Contemporary Rhinoplasty

Edited by Sebastian Torres Farr

Published in London, United Kingdom

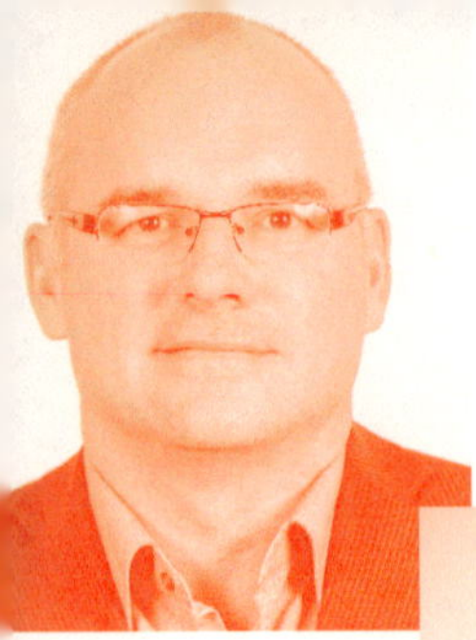
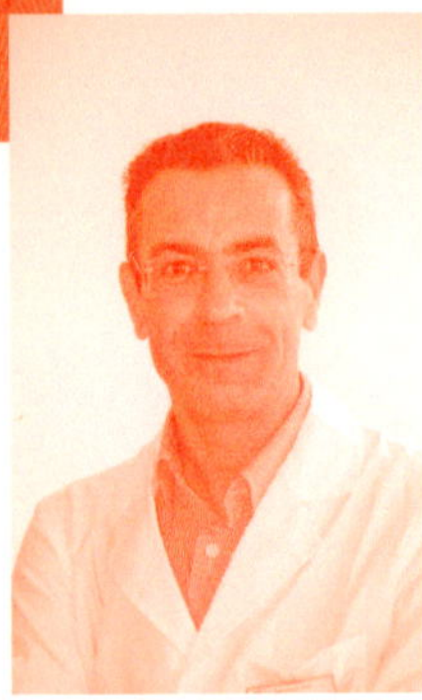
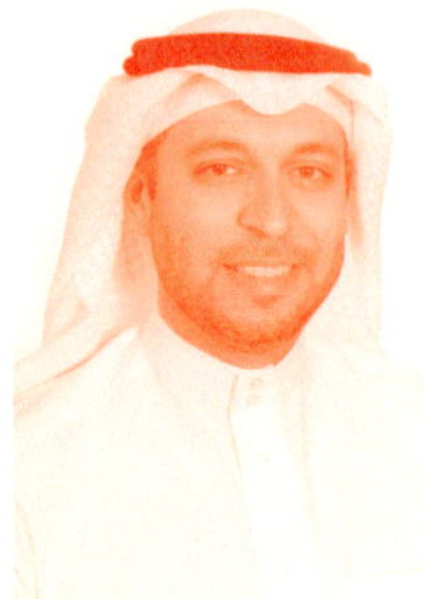
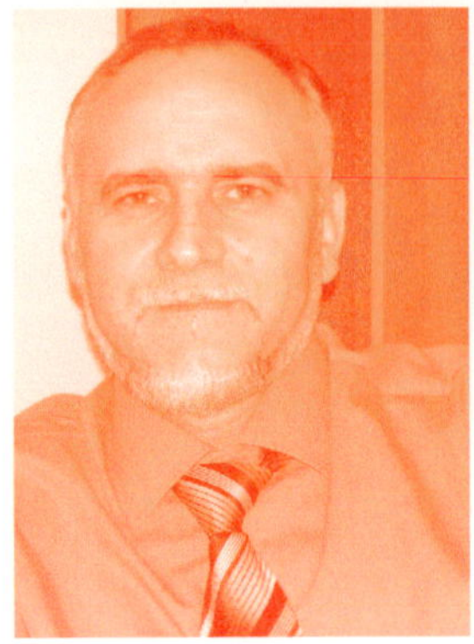
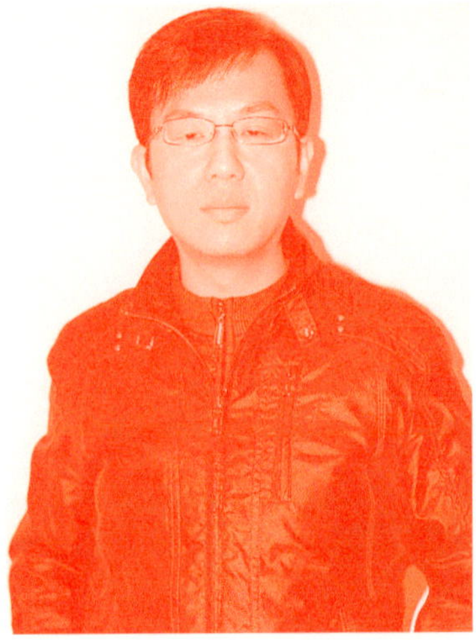
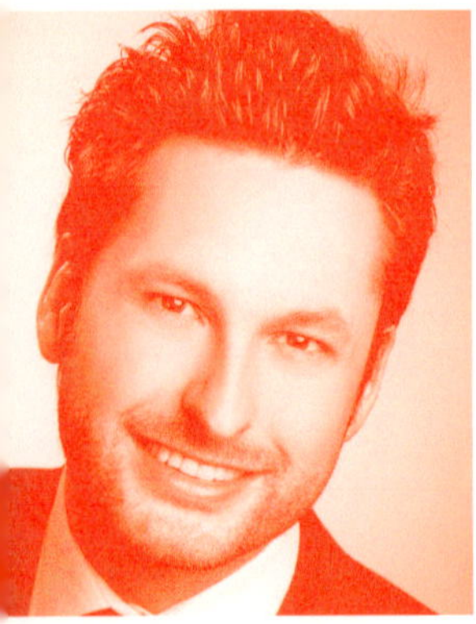
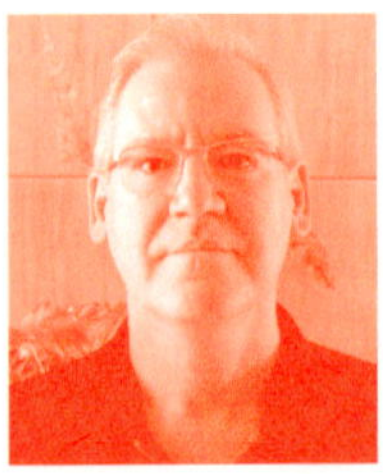

IntechOpen

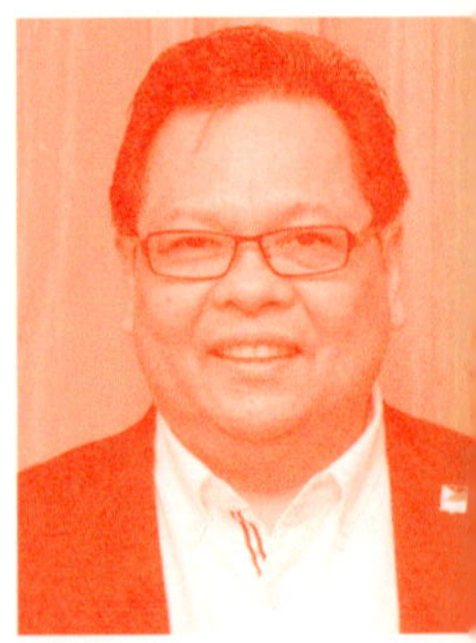
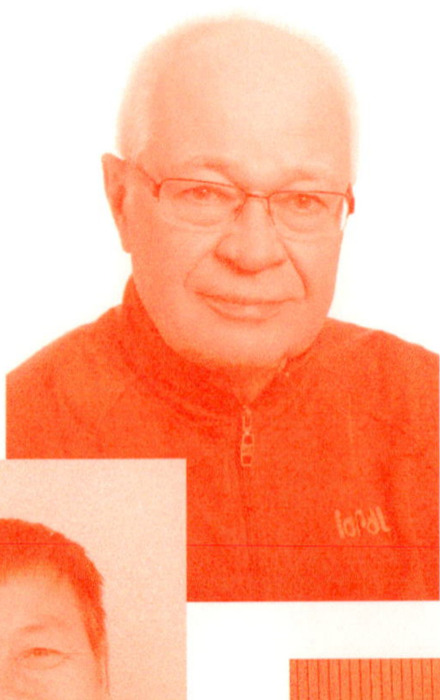
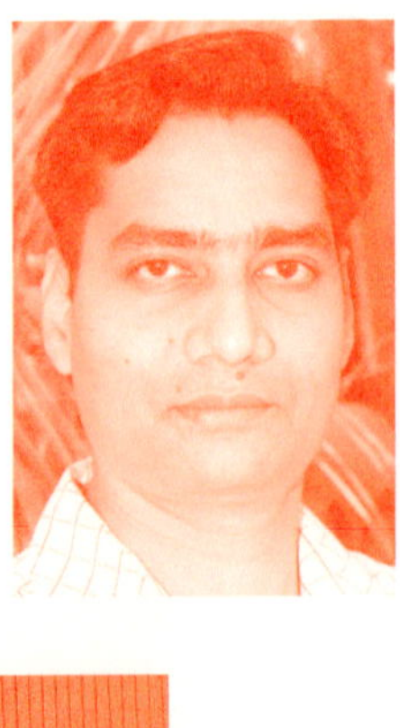
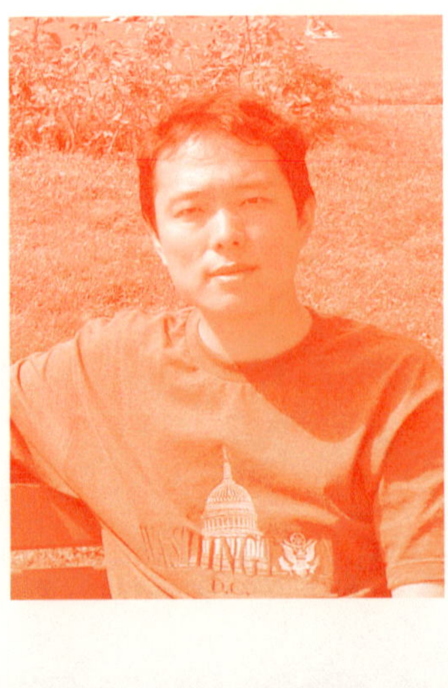
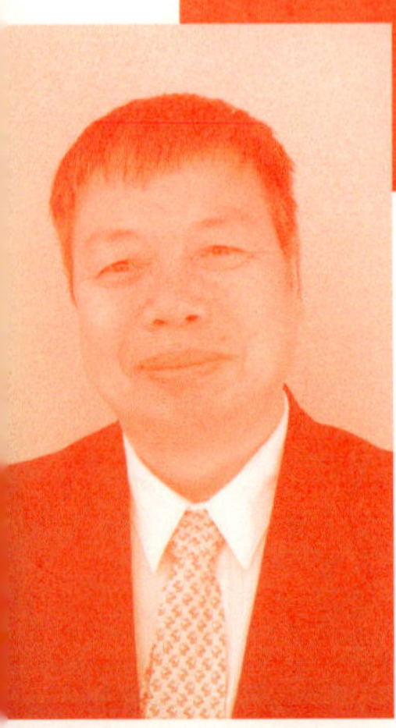
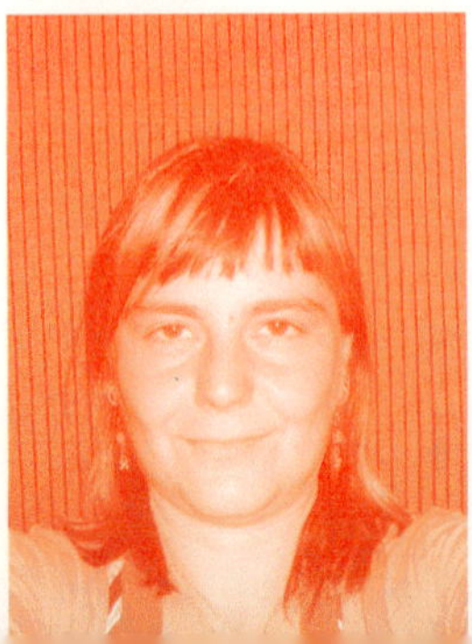

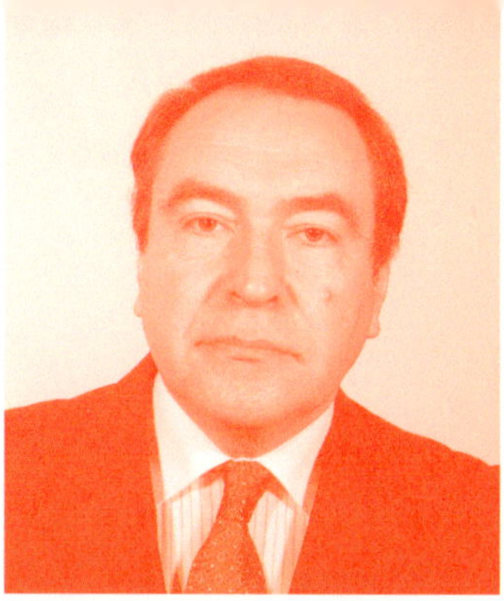
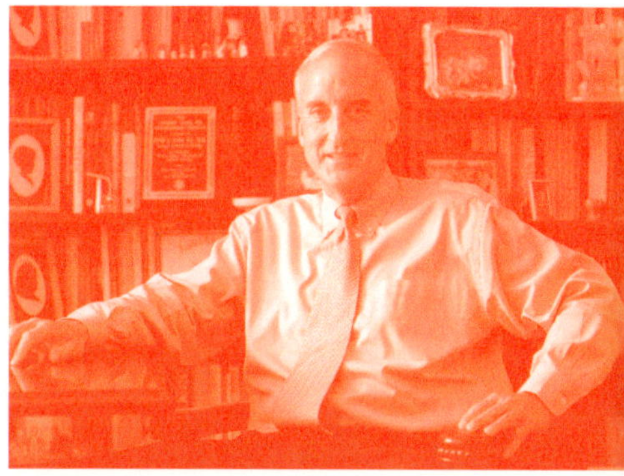
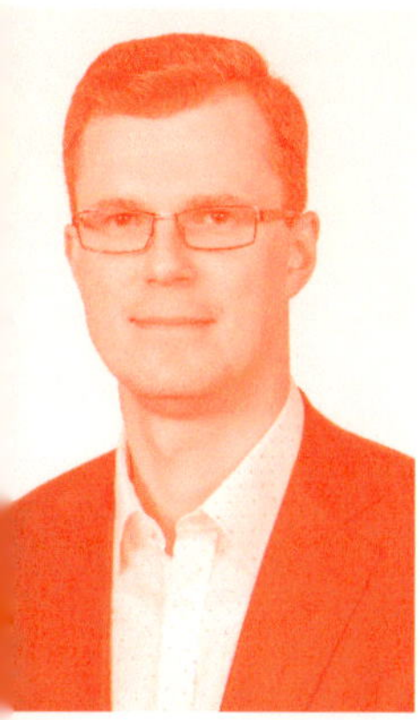
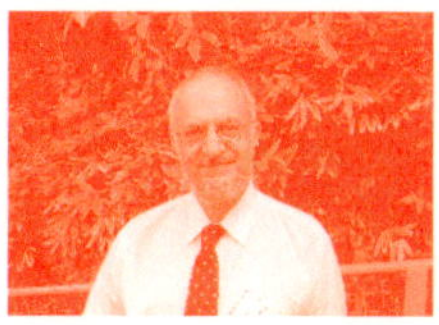
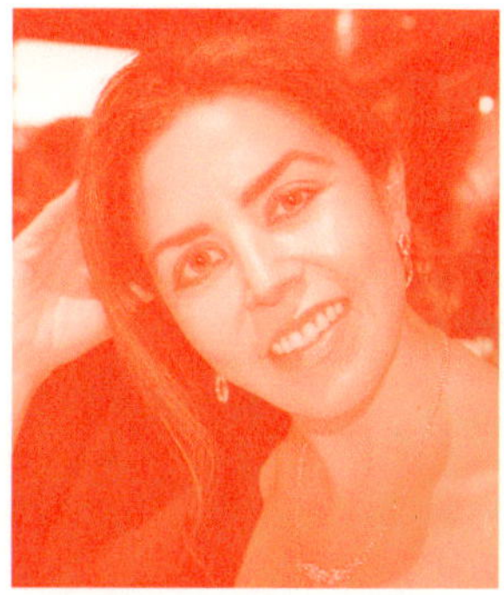

Supporting open minds since 2005

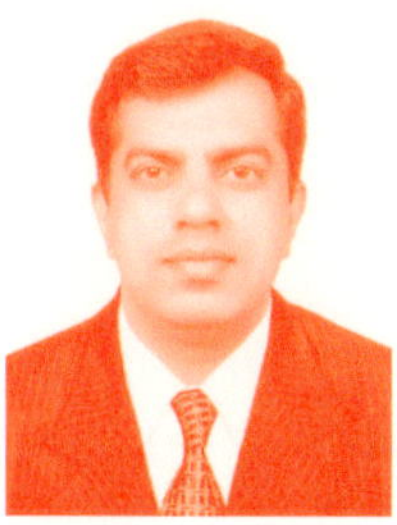
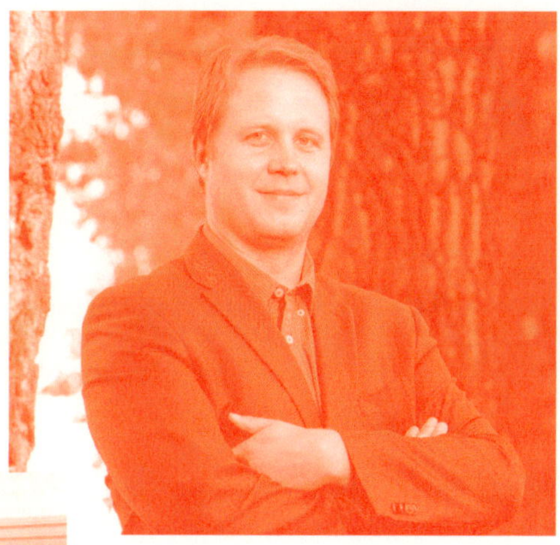
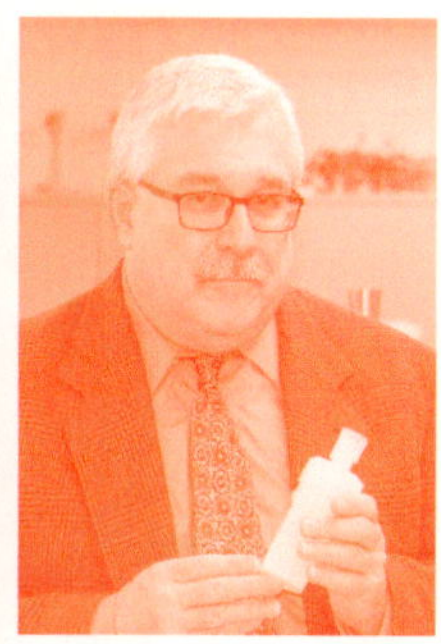
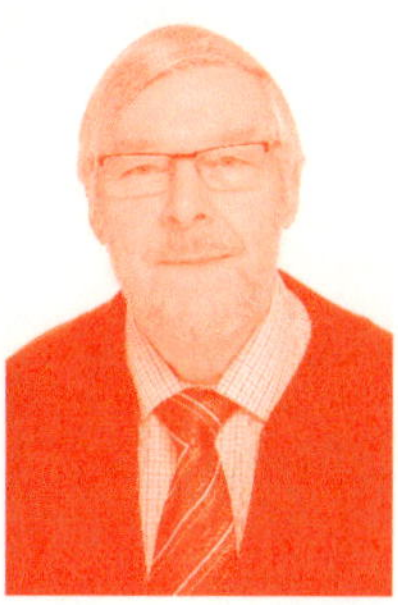
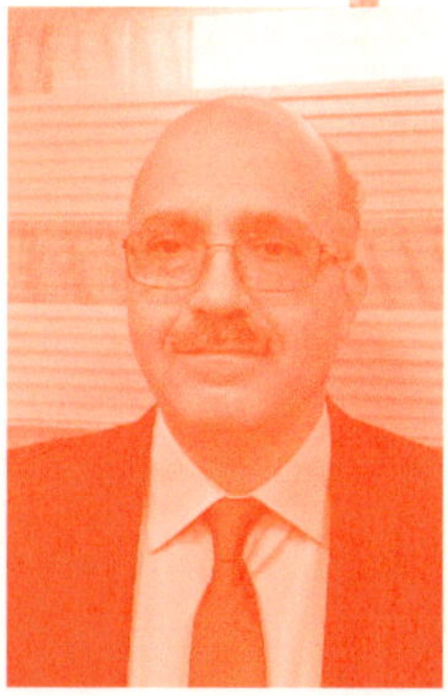
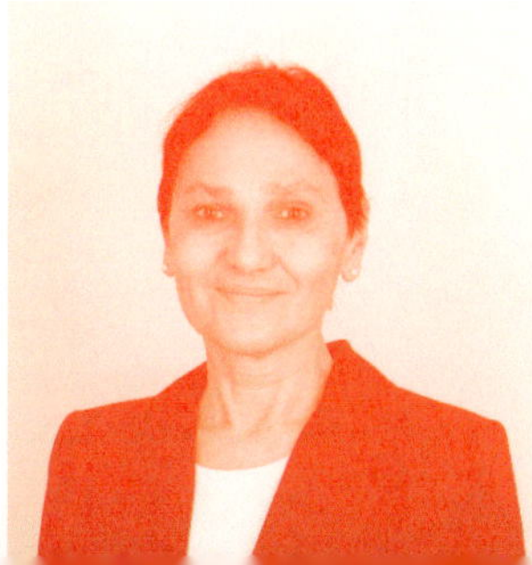
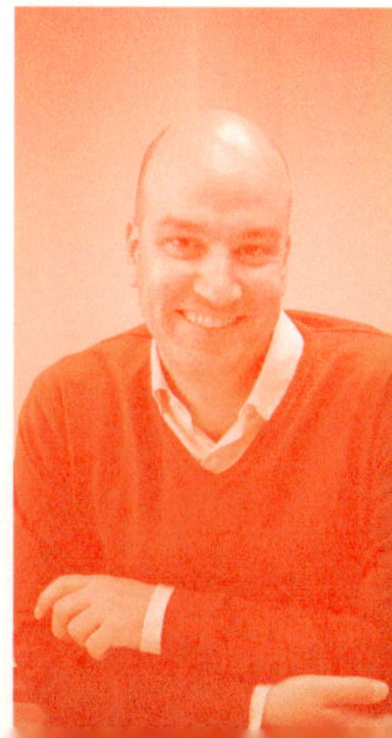

Contemporary Rhinoplasty
http://dx.doi.org/10.5772/intechopen.79209
Edited by Sebastian Torres Farr

Contributors
Aditya Yeolekar, Ken-Ichi Hisamatsu, Norhafiza Mat Lazim, Giacomo Spinato, Paolo Boscolo Rizzo Paolo Boscolo Rizzo, Tito Marianetti, Angelo Cuzalina, Ahmed Tamim, Wenceslao M Calonge, Daniel Espinoza Kauer, Diana Oesch Ortiz, Pedro S. Arquero, Sebastian Torres Farr

First published in London, United Kingdom, 2019 by IntechOpen
IntechOpen is the global imprint of INTECHOPEN LIMITED, registered in England and Wales, registration number: 11086078, 7th floor, 10 Lower Thames Street, London, EC3R 6AF, United Kingdom
Printed in Croatia

British Library Cataloguing-in-Publication Data
A catalogue record for this book is available from the British Library

Additional hard and PDF copies can be obtained from orders@intechopen.com

Contemporary Rhinoplasty
Edited by Sebastian Torres Farr
p. cm.
Print ISBN 978-1-83968-027-4
Online ISBN 978-1-83968-028-1
eBook (PDF) ISBN 978-1-83968-029-8

For EU product safety concerns:
IN TECH d.o.o., Prolaz Marije Krucifikse Kozulić 3, 51000 Rijeka, Croatia, info@intechopen.com or visit our website at intechopen.com.

Meet the editor

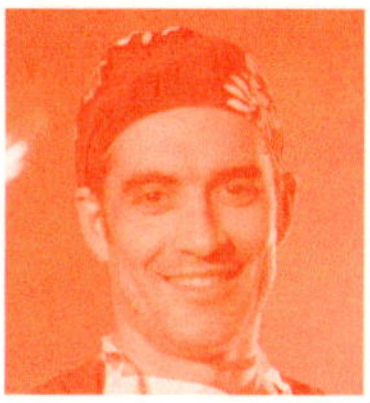

Dr. Torres is fully committed to achieving excellence, having trained himself in North and South America, Europe, and Asia. He achieved a double degree MD in Chile and Italy, and obtained a specialty in cranio-maxillofacial surgery at Messina University, Italy. He completed his Master's degree in Aesthetic Medicine, Dentofacial Abnormalities, Open Rhinoplasty, and Breast Reconstruction. Dr. Torres has attended more than 50 masterclasses and cadaver dissections courses and published more than 30 international articles. In 2010 he was awarded by EACMFS as one of the most talented young surgeons in Europe. He works as the main aesthetic plastic surgeon and clinical director in the Cirugia 360 Clinic in Santiago, Chile. Dr. Torres is also an inventor, having patented different devices in the field of aesthetic surgery. He is interested in teaching and giving courses and seminars worldwide.

Contents

Preface

It is with great pleasure that I introduce to you this new rhinoplasty book, which will update a number of areas regarding nasal surgery. The panel of authors is formed by highly talented and worldwide recognized rhinoplasty surgeons. Among the book content the novel surgeon will surely appreciate the overview of nasal aesthetics, correct diagnosis and treatment planning, as well as the surgical learning curve chapter. Clinical management and surgical decision protocol in saddle nose deformity are also discussed. Technical pitfalls on alar rim grafts as part of our surgical armamentarium are highlighted. Moreover, the combination of the procedure in concomitancy with morbid conditions such as sleep breathing disorders, clefts, and head and neck cancer are presented. Whatever your expertise in rhinoplasty the book will add something to your practice and enhance your future procedures.

Sebastian Torres Farr
Torres Aesthetic Clinic,
Chile

Section 1

Introduction

Chapter 1

Introductory Chapter: Nasal Aesthetics, Defining a Correct Diagnosis and Treatment Planning

Elmer Sebastian Torres Farr

1. Nasal aesthetics

Beauty is a condition that is always admired by masses. For that reason, great interest has been given into finding a common denominator that would allow to establish and define a setting to evaluate, replicate and improve this character.

From antiquity, beauty has tried to be defined through anthropometric, planimetric and esthereometric measurements. The truth is that beauty has always been hard to measure due to intrinsic subjectivity within it.

Beauty is associated with youth, health and strength in nature, all valuable features for survival in the animal kingdom.

Facial beauty has objective parameters that are related to mathematics (angles and heights) and subjective perceptions that are automatic and innate [1]. The observer defines within seconds if what they look is attractive or not. The former causes that to define beauty we shall combine science and art.

Facial beauty is a combination of features that should be harmonic, defined, balanced, elevated, symmetric, characteristic and in volumetric proportion. Each face is unique, and as such the difference between a normal and a beautiful face differs in a few millimetres or angular degrees.

Facial traits differ in importance order, being the nose at the intermediate level behind the eyes, eyebrow, cheekbones and lips. Nevertheless, the nose being at the centre of the face connects all the elements together and allows the eye of the beholder to flow in a complete facial beauty perception or to stay trapped in isolated components categorised as beautiful [2].

A beautiful nose is defined as:

- Straight or slight concave dorsum
- Moderate nasofrontal angle at radix
- Mild width bony pyramid
- Good tip projection/rotation
- Parallel aesthetic dorsal lines
- Length proportional to facial height

2. Defining a correct diagnosis

Nasal aesthetics, although with experience is instantly evaluated by the surgeon at consultation, at first must be incorporated in a schematised protocol of photograph analysis to assist the professional to achieve a correct diagnosis that will command a related correction and satisfactory outcome [3].

The consultation should start with complete nasal history, taking into consideration aesthetic and functional disorders. Previous nasal aesthetic procedures such as dermal fillers, lasers and others should be promptly recorded as they may alter the surgical result.

The use of dermal fillers, nowadays widely spread, merits special attention as some of them may be dissolved prior to the surgery (hyaluronic acid), while others are more difficult to eliminate (hydroxyapatite, polycaprolactone). Some may compromise vascularisation and skin viability, and removal may be difficult or impossible (silicone, polymethylmethacrylate) [4].

Previous nasal surgeries must be clarified as they may provoke scarring and inflammation and reduce potential cartilage graft availability.

An initial physical nasal exam should be performed including external and internal morphology with both aesthetic and functional assessments.

Imaging should be the subsequent step in the correct case recording, through conventional or 3D imaging devices (3D LifeViz, QuantifiCare, Paris, France). The former will allow detailed nasal mathematical analysis that will be balanced with clinical impression and patients' requests to obtain a final treatment plan.

The measurements of distances and angles are suitable to be done with basic printed photographs and pencils or with more modern software and calibrated distances. The latter allow impressive virtual surgery simulations that may shorten the distance between the patient wishes and surgeons' understanding (**Figure 1**).

Nasal Anatomic Examination

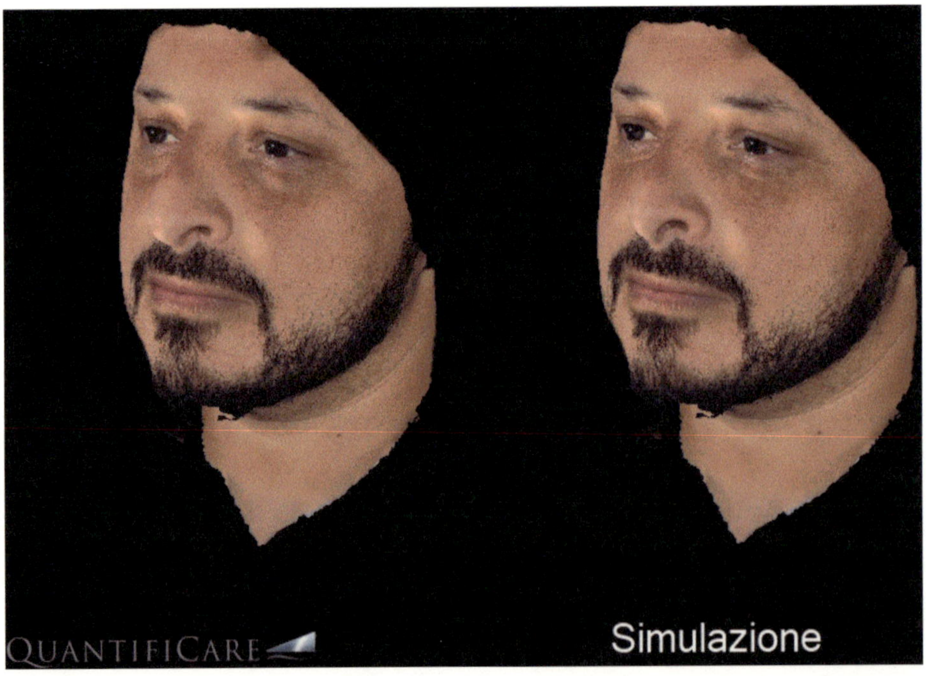

Figure 1.
Virtual rhinoplasty 3D morphing treatment plan.

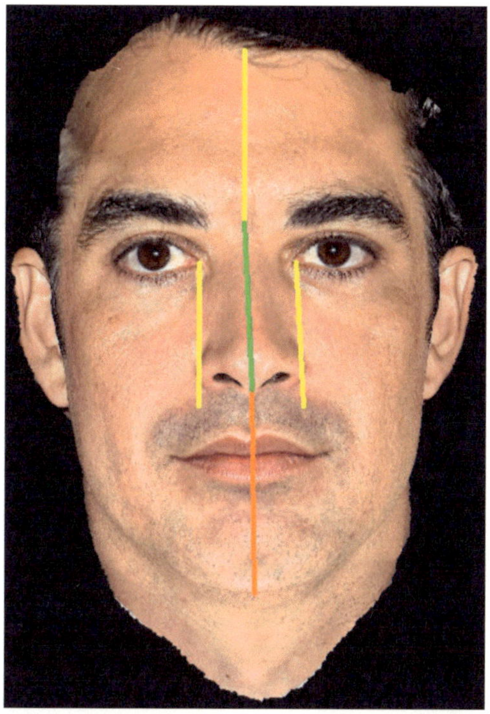

Figure 2.
Facial thirds and (upper, middle, lower) nose width. The latter should be within the vertical lines that descend from the inner canthus.

- **Facial Proportions** (mm) (**Figure 2**):
  - **Upper**:
  - **Middle**:
  - **Lower**: (*Maxilla*, *Occlusion*, *Chin*)
  Vertical: Normal/ Excess / Deficit
  Anterior/Posterior: Normal/ Retrusion/Protrusion

- **Skin:** Normal/Thick/Thin Phototype: Scars:

- **Dorsum:**

  - **Ideal Nasal Length** (Radix to Tip -RT) = 0,67 x MFH (Midfacial height) ➔ GB (Glabella)- ABP (Alar Base Plane)
  - **Radix**: Projection (from Corneal Plane): RT x 0,28 (9-14mm Average 11mm) Normal /Low/ High
  -**Nasofrontal Angle**: (115-130 °, Average 120 °) (**Figure 3**)
  -**Height**: Hump +/- Bony/Cartilage
  -**Width**: Dorsal Aesthetic Lines Symmetric / Asymmetric / Deviation L/R
  -**Other:**

- **Tip:**
  -Projection (from Alar Crease- AC) = 0,67x RT
  -Domes Shape: Normal/ Bulbous/ Boxy/ Pinch
  -Columellar-Lobular Angle (30-45 °) (**Figure 3**)
  -Columellar-Lip Angle (100-115 ° ♀ / 90-105 ° ♂) (**Figure 3**)
  -Other:

- **Base (Figure 4):**
  -Columellar Lobule Ratio: (2/1)
  -Nostrils: Shape /Symmetry Normal/ Hanging/ Retracted
  - Columella: Normal/ Hanging/ Retracted
  - Alar Width: (Inner Canthus-IC to IC) Normal/ Augmented/ Reduced

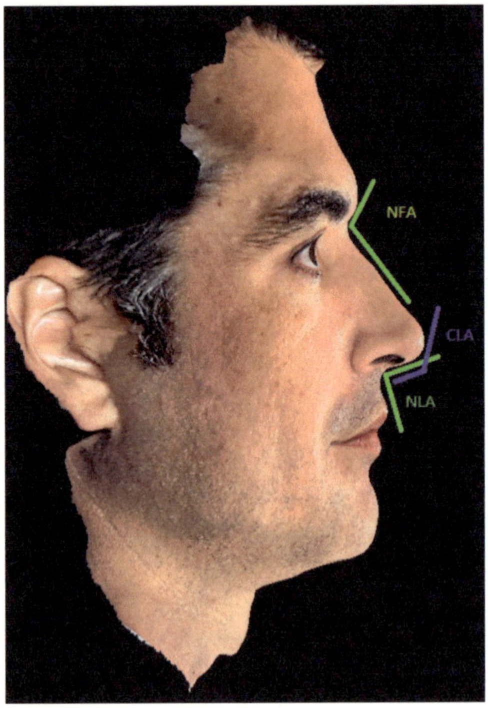

Figure 3.
Nasal angles. NFA, nasofrontal angle. NLA, nasolabial angle, CLA, columellar lobular angle.

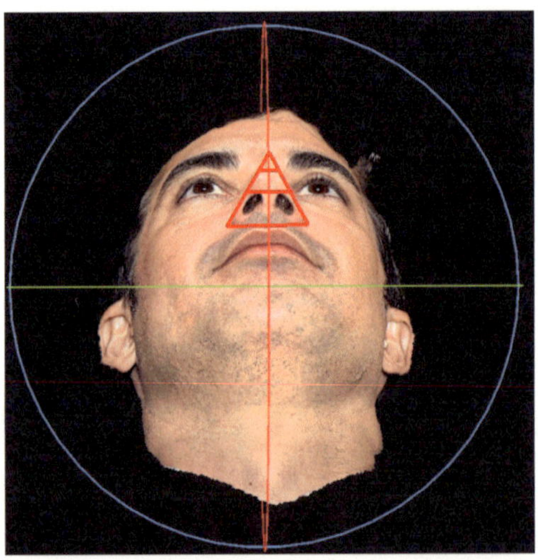

Figure 4.
Nasal base. The equilateral triangle that forms should be centred, symmetrical and well projected. The distance between the base of the columella and anterior portion of the nostrils should be 2/3 of the total distance to the nose tip.

- **Functionality**
  - External valves: Competent / Incompetent L/R
  - Internal valves: Permeable / Impermeable L/R
  - Rhinomanometry:
  - CT Scan:

- **Mathematical Diagnosis:**

- **Clinical Diagnosis:**

3. Treatment planning

Taking into consideration patient requests or goals, physician first impression and priorities and mathematical analysis, a surgical plan is elaborated. The idea is to have everything set before starting the surgical corrections. Step by step actions are intended to avoid or reduce last minute surprises or improvisation [5].

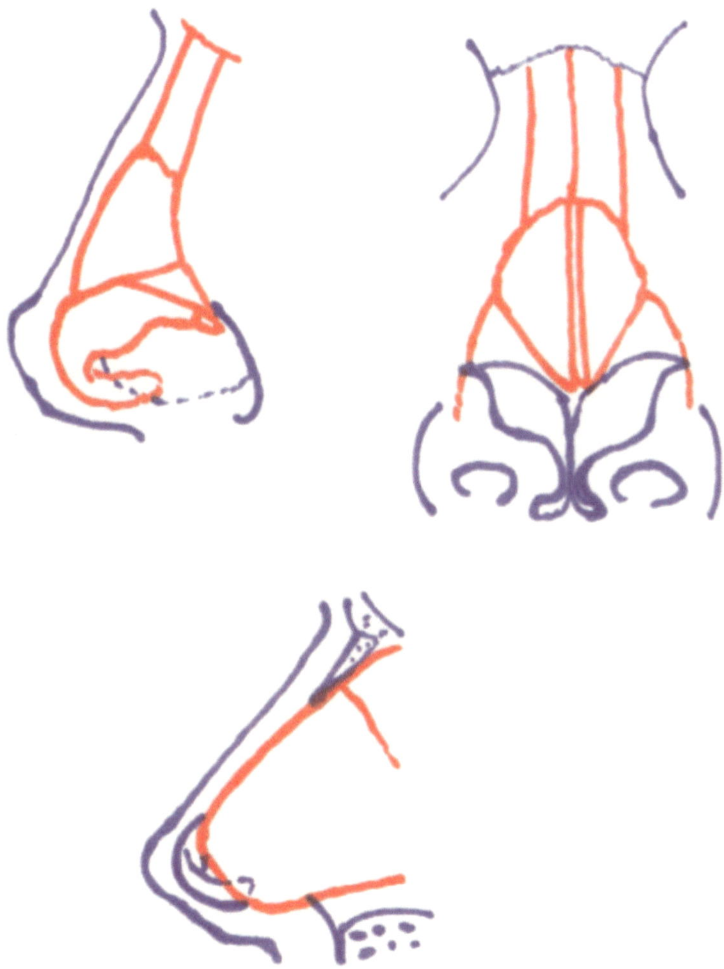

Figure 5.
Surgical plan. All surgical steps should be recorded in this record for better surgical planning and future control and outcome analysis.

Where and what incision should be placed, what corrections are a must, and in what order are they going to be performed? What materials would we need to build the internal framework (grafts)? Which are going to be harvesting sites? The idea is to answer every question in the surgeon's head up front.

To think, to feel and then to perform, that is the safest way to approach rhinoplasty and reduce the revision rate.

- **Surgical Plan** (**Figure** 5)
  - Patient main goals *(3)*:
  -Rhinoplasty Primary / Secondary
  - Incisions and approach: Transcollumellar/ Other Closed / Open
  - Nasal Tip: Rotate / Under rotate Project / Deproject Reduce /Augment (width)
  -Dorsum: Augment / Reduce / Smooth
  -Dorsal Aesthetic Lines: Define / Deviate L/R
  -Oshteotomies: Lateral / Transverse / Medial / Continuous Deviate L/R
  -Alar Base/ Nostril/ Anterior Nasal Spine Reduction / Augmentation
  - Functional: External Valves Correction +/- Internal Valve Correction +/-
  - Grafts Needed: Name and Draw
  -Graft Harvest Area: Septum / Conchae / Rib
  -Other:
  -Difficulty (1-10)
  -Estimated time:

Author details

Elmer Sebastian Torres Farr
Maxillofacial, Plastic and Aesthetic Surgery, Private Practice, Santiago, Chile

*Address all correspondence to: storres100@gmail.com

References

[1] Vucinic N, Tubbs S, Eric M, et al. What do we find attractive about the face?: Survey study with application to aesthetic surgery. Clinical Anatomy. 24 Aug 2019. DOI: 10.1002/ca.23455

[2] Panfilov DE. Aesthetic Surgery of the Facial Mosaic. Berlin, Germany: Springer; 2007

[3] Rohrich RJ. Dallas Rhinoplasty: Nasal Surgery by the Masters. 3rd ed. Dallas, USA: CRC Press; 2014

[4] Kalantar Motamedi MH. Chapter 30: A textbook of advanced oral and maxillo facial surgery. In: Torres S, Marianetti T, editors. Management of Common Complications in Rhinoplasty and Medical Rhinoplasty. Vol. 3. Croatia: IntechOpen; 2016

[5] Daniel RK. Mastering Rhinoplasty: A Comprehensive Atlas of Surgical Techniques with Integrated Video Clips. USA: Springer Nature; 2009

Section 2

Preoperatory Considerations

Chapter 2

Learning Curve and Septorhinoplasty

Aditya Yeolekar

Abstract

The learning curve as a concept has been considered and discussed in medical education and surgical practice. Rollin Daniel stated that rhinoplasty is the most difficult of all cosmetic operations for three reasons: (a) nasal anatomy is highly variable, (b) the procedure must correct form and function and (c) patients' expectations. With this in mind, a study was planned on learning curve in septorhinoplasty based on a surgeon questionnaire. The aims of the study were to extract the idea of learning curve from different surgeons across experience about septorhioplasty, to calculate certain parameters of the learning curve in rhinoplasty and to prepare a roadmap for an early rhinoplasty surgeon. The conclusion derived from the study was the concept of the learning curve in rhinoplasty should not be generalised as certain factors, for example, minimum number to achieve proficiency has a wide range. *It is thought that each type of rhinoplasty should be dealt with separately and learning curve calculated accordingly. A roadmap for a novice surgeon is hereby charted out.*

Keywords: the learning curve, septorhinoplasty

1. Introduction

The concept of the learning curve was first described in 1885 by Hermann Ebbinghaus (**Figure 1**). It is a graphical representation, where the vertical axis depicts increase in learning as compared to the horizontal axis that suggests experience. It is also referred to as experience curve and productivity curve. In medical terms it can now be described as improvement in one's technical performance over time secondary to increased experience and training [1-5].

The learning curve in surgical procedure (**Figure 2**) has four phases: Phase I is commencement of training—residency (post-graduation, senior residency). Phase II is a stepwise ascent in which individuals' performance improves, and this may take a lot of time (fellowship programme, working at a high-volume centre and working under a senior mentor). Phase III is when a procedure is performed independently and with competence (medical university and private practice). This is followed by a plateau where experience improves progress by only smaller fractions. This is followed by a downward sloping curve due to advancing age.

Therefore, a study was formulated which would help to plan a learning curve in the speciality of septorhinoplasty.

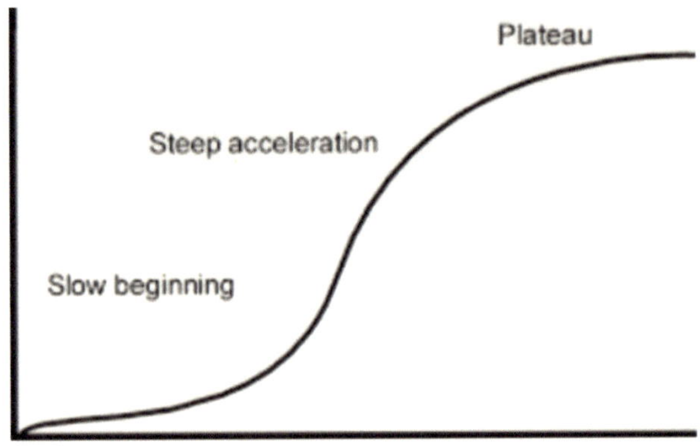

Figure 1.
The learning curve.

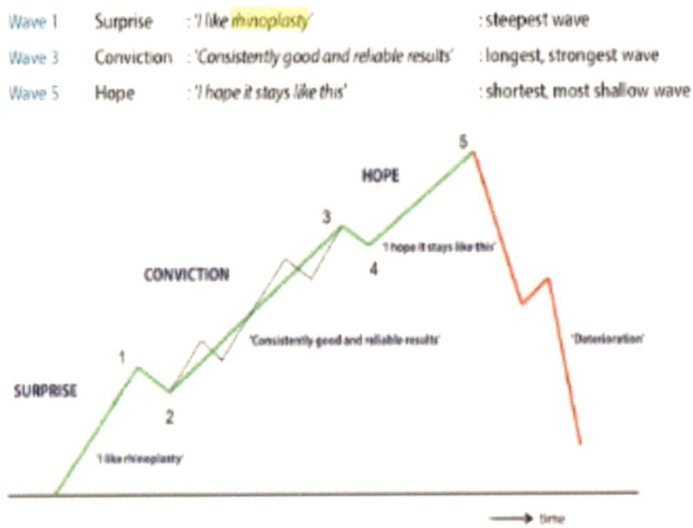

Figure 2.
A surgical learning curve.

1.1 Aims

1. To extract the learning curve of rhinoplasty from surgeons across a spectrum of experience (less experienced to experienced).

2. To calculate the learning curve in rhinoplasty as for other surgical procedures, that is, minimum number of procedures to attain proficiency, surgical time and accelerators to your learning curve.

3. To suggest a roadmap for early career rhinoplasty surgeon.

1.2 Methodology

A clinical-based questionnaire was prepared. The study was executed at a workshop attended by rhinoplasty surgeons around the globe. It was completely

Group	No. of open rhinoplasties performed	Number of surgeons
A	0–10	6
B	11–100	11
C	101–500	7
D	More than 500	6

Table 1.
Surgeon group.

Group	Range	Mean
A (0–10)	75–100	86.66
B (11–100)	25–80	48.18
C (101–500)	20–100	65.71
D (more than 500)	50–200	108.33

Table 2.
Minimum number of surgeries required to achieve proficiency.

Accelerator	Mean
Cadaveric dissection (self)	8.06
Cadaveric dissection (observe)	5.79
Attending workshop/conference	8.1
Analysis of own cases (self)	8.26
Analysis of own cases (expert colleague)	8.6
Writing article/publication	5.1
Observership under expert	9.66
Structured fellowship	9.43
Total no. of rhinoplasties	9.56

Table 3.
Learning curve accelerators.

voluntary, and no personal details pertaining to name and place of practice were obtained. Seventy questionnaires were distributed. A total of 30 completely filled questionnaires were obtained and further analysed.

1.3 Observations and results

A total of 30 surgeons participated that included resident surgeons, assistant surgeons, specialist surgeons and private practitioners (plastic/ENT/maxillofacial). It was found that exclusive open rhinoplasty was practised by 20 surgeons whereas open and closed by 10 surgeons.

The participants were distributed into four groups according to the level of experience (**Table 1**).

The lowest number was 0 (resident doctor) and the highest was 3000.

The number of procedures required to achieve proficiency in open rhinoplasty was studied (**Table 2**).

This emphasised that surgeons with lesser experience thought about 86 procedures are to be dealt with to achieve proficiency (i.e. the operation is difficult). The mid-level thought the figure in the range of 48–65 procedures to achieve proficiency. The masters with more experience inarguably stated minimum 100 procedures are required to achieve proficiency. This once again implied the intricacies and complexities of the surgery.

Change in operation time as surgical experience increases was studied. All the four groups thought that as experience grows, one can perform the procedure earlier by about 60 min.

Learning curve accelerators are methods by which one can accelerate the learning curve. Participants were asked to rate the importance of each on a scale of 0–10 (10 being most important) (**Table 3**).

2. Conclusion

The minimum number of procedures required to achieve proficiency in open rhinoplasty ranged from 20 to 100 with mean of 76.66 and in closed rhinoplasty from 40 to 200 with mean of 106. It was uniformly opined that as experience grows the surgical time of the procedure reduces by about an hour. The most important accelerators of learning were observership under an expert, well-structured fellowship and number of procedures one performs.

3. Discussion

The surgery of septorhinoplasty is difficult to understand even with adequate knowledge because it relies on understanding the various expectations the patient has and the act of delivering consistent results. The surgical techniques used by different surgeons are unique and sometimes not reproducible. It being a highly individualised surgery, no single technique works all the time. A good photographic analysis helps one to prepare a surgical plan be it structural rhinoplasty or a surface rhinoplasty. It surgical procedure addresses various issues: dorsal hump, dorsal deviation, tip, radix and other deformities. The surgical time remains static over one's career or even increases a little by experience in doing additional graft work. Factors like temperament and personality of surgeon might also affect the results. According to W. Gubisch, one can become a good rhinoplasty surgeon only if one can address the nasal septum effectively. In his book on *Advanced Caucasian and Mediterranean Rhinoplasty*, P.J.F.M. Lohius stated that the learning curve depends on genes, exercise and also on luck [6]. Senior Surgeon Rollin Daniel has described few accelerators, namely, detailed preoperative analysis of photos in various view, well-written surgical workflow, use of instruments of good-quality, intraoperative photography and self-explanatory diagrams, analysis of postoperative photos, revision surgeries of own patients, reading the subject, attending meetings for paper presentations and publishing articles [7].

The formulated path in septorhinoplasty:

A. To learn good photography techniques in standardised angles using good lens (macro/telephoto) with standard lighting environment.

B. To perform self-analysis of patients' preoperative photographs and devise a plan of surgery.

C. The single most important point is the correct diagnosis of the deformity so that there are no surprises during surgery.

D. To discuss your plan or roadmap of surgery with master, mentor or chief operative surgeon.

E. To assist more than 100 cases of septorhinoplasty as a first assistant both in open and closed rhinoplasty techniques and. to attend to postoperative care and protocols.

F. To independently perform functional septoplasty or submucous resection of septum, minimum of 100 procedures, to understand septal anatomy better and also perform pre-operative nasal endoscopy to understand intranasal anatomy mainly inferior turbinates and posterior septum.

G. To watch live operations by experts and surgical videos by stalwarts.

H. To perform cadaver dissections.

I. One can use plastic or cardboard cutouts in form of different grafts for practice during cadaveric dissections.

J. To classify cases according to difficulty, that is, easy, intermediate and difficult rhinoplasty.

K. In difficult rhinoplasty cases, one should not hesitate to involve another experienced colleague in the surgery.

Cases to be avoided by rhinoplasty surgeon of experience of less than 10 cases are extracorporeal septoplasty, tip plasty, cleft nose, extreme bony deviations, saddle nose, revision cases, pure aesthetic, ethnic nose, multiple deformities and unrealistic expectations. Cases to be avoided by surgeon with experience of more than 10 but less than 100 rhinoplasties are saddle nose, cleft nose, ethnic nose, revision cases and secondary skinny nose.

L. To follow surgical techniques of one mentor repeatedly over 100 operations, improvised with each operation. To incorporate inputs from other surgeons and device your own plan for each subtype of rhinoplasty.

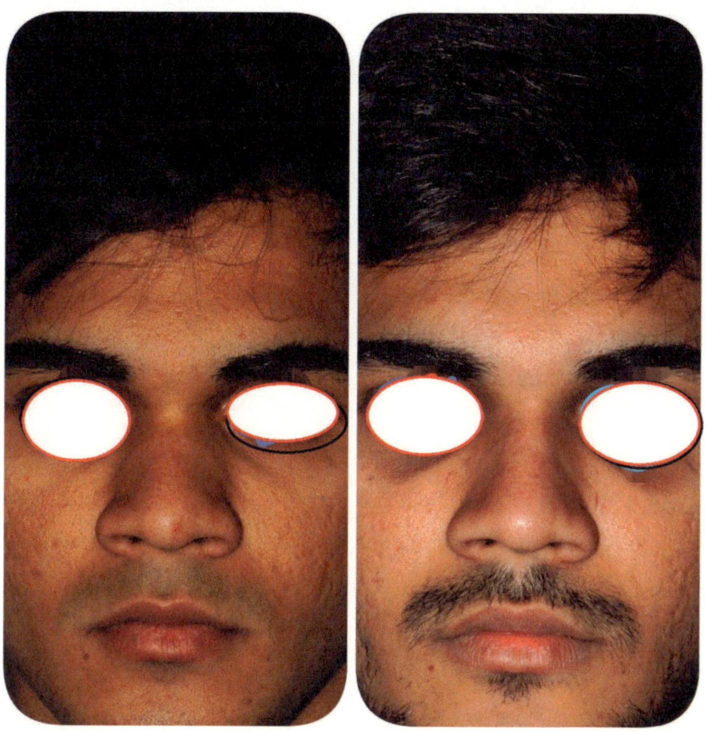

Figure 3.
Simple case 1: wide dorsum.

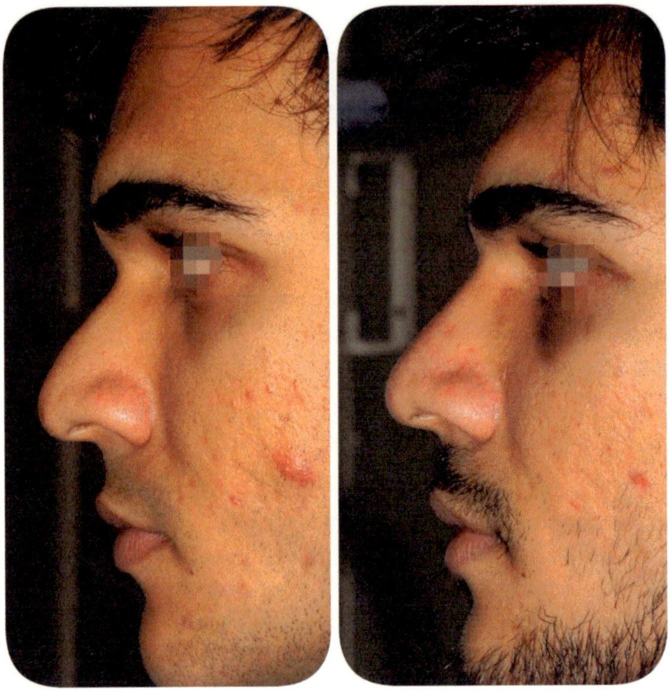

Figure 4.
Simple case 1: correction of deep radix with free diced cartilage.

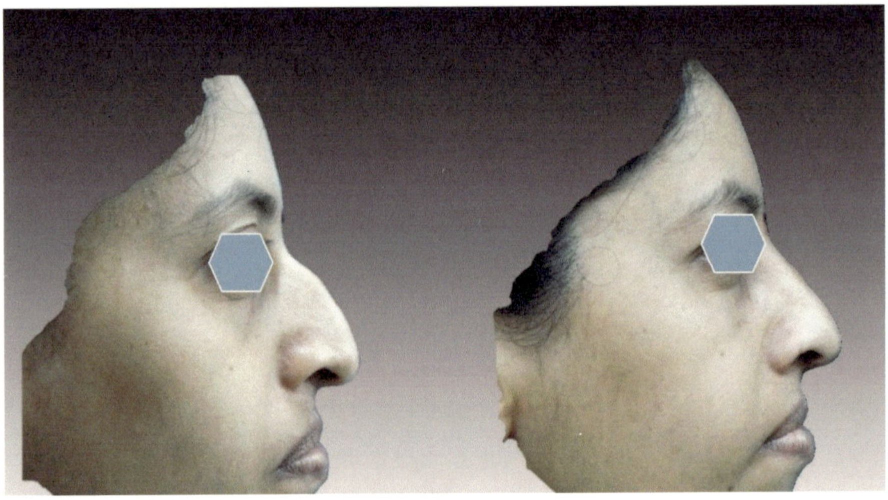

Figure 5.
Simple case 2: hump nose. Here what would have been better is a supratip break.

M. To present one's work at various conferences at local, national and international fora.

N. To periodically visit various centres around the globe to understand and update oneself about finer nuances of open and closed rhinoplasty.

In my honest opinion, one should assist a rhinoplasty surgeon for a minimum 25 cases along with cadaveric dissections and attending courses at established centres around the globe, like the ones at Stuttgart, Bergamo, Milan, Chicago, London, Singapore and the European and American congresses.

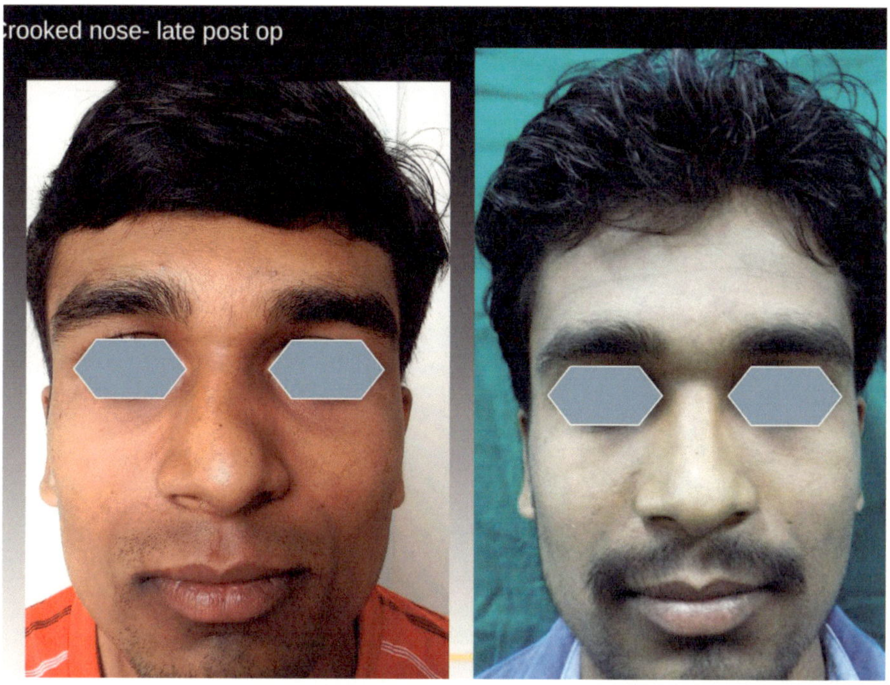

Figure 6.
Intermediate 1: crooked nose with bulbous tip.

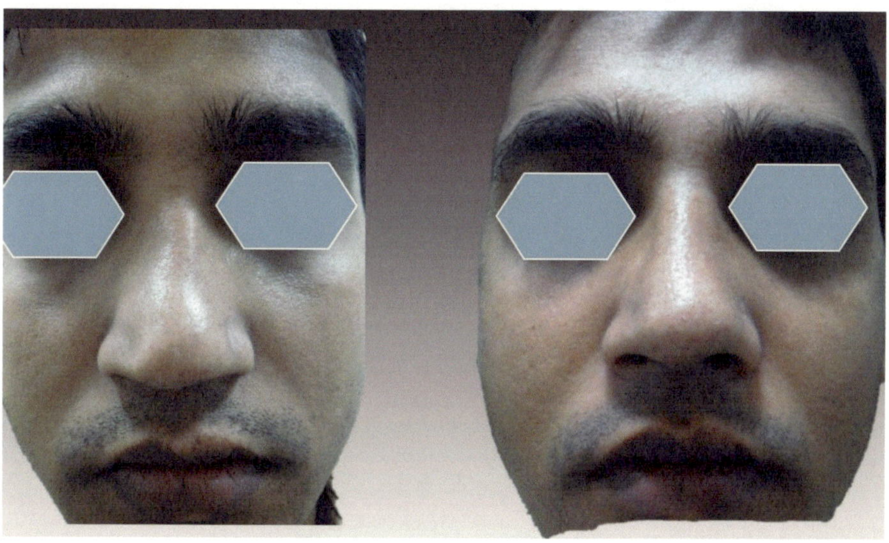

Figure 7.
Intermediate 2: crooked nose with ptotic tip.

This should be followed by doing simple cases in presence of your mentor or an experienced surgeon (**Figures 3** and **4**).

A long-term follow-up of cases should be maintained, and photographic analysis should be compared to pre-op at 6 months and yearly interval. This should be discussed with your senior colleague who shall criticise a point out your mistakes.

This shall help you to undertake intermediate difficult surgeries as follows:

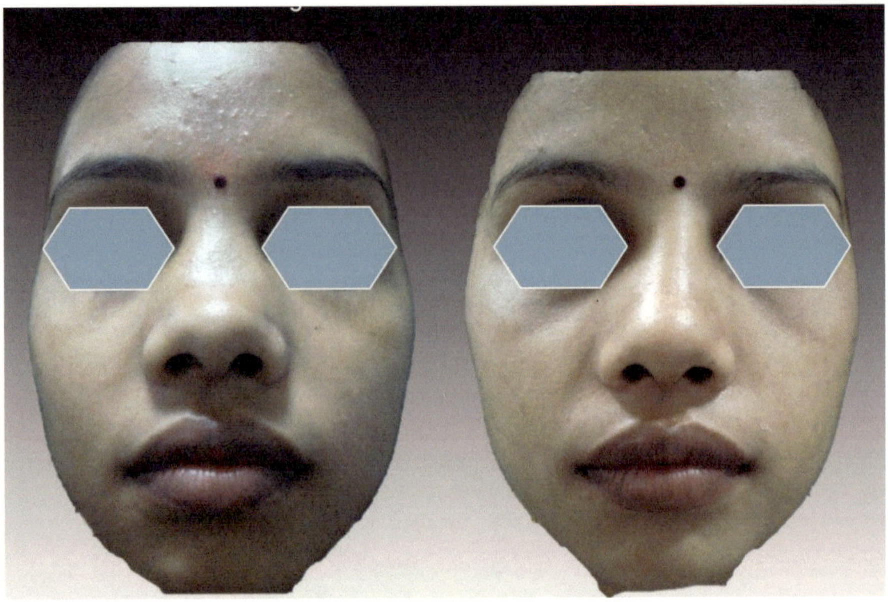

Figure 8.
Intermediate 3: saddle nose. Repair with costal cartilage.

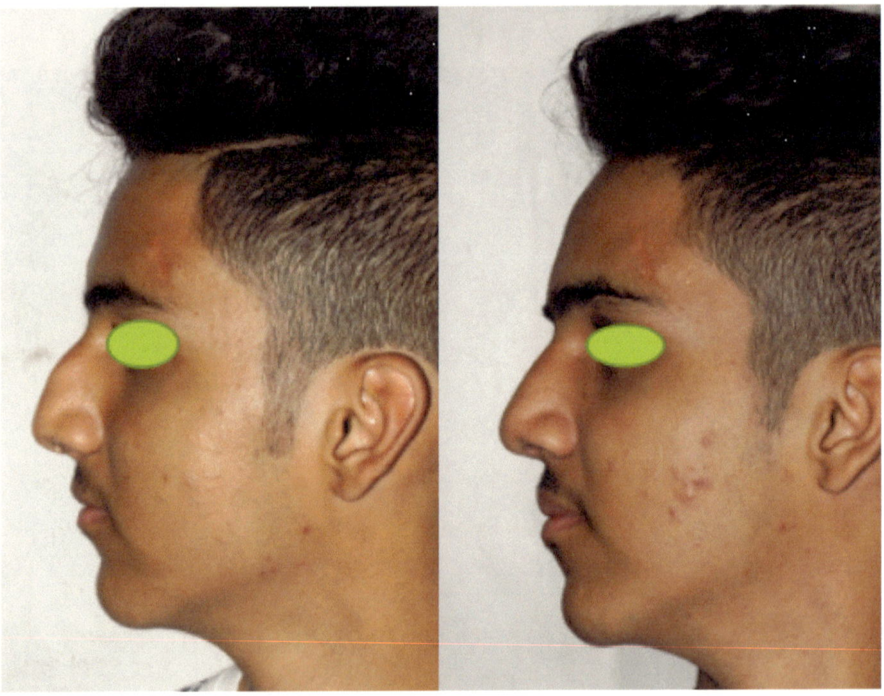

Figure 9.
Difficult 1: crooked nose with hump with deviated nasal septum.

This refines your surgery in a better way. Also never hesitate to ask for help from seniors as they themselves have been through similar phases and only they can guide you better rather than being lost (**Figures 5–8**).

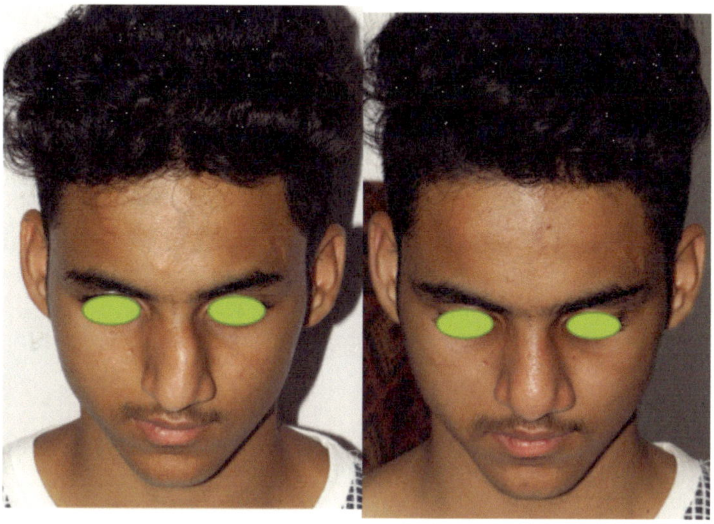

Figure 10.
Difficult 1: requiring extracorporeal septoplasty approach.

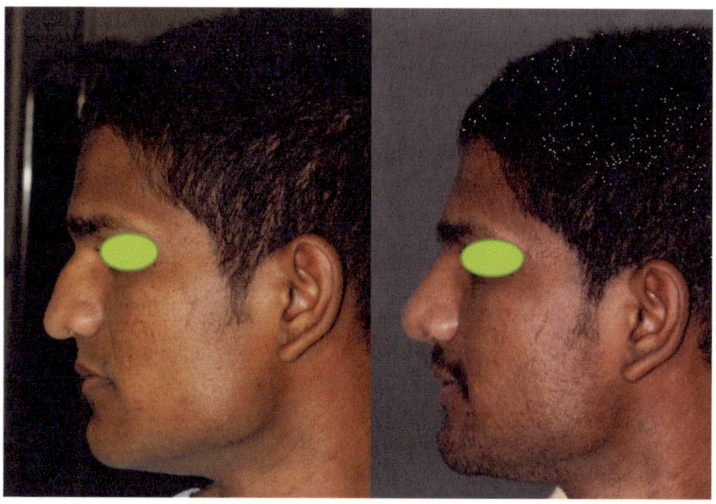

Figure 11.
Difficult 2: deep radix, wide dorsum with ptotic tip. Extracorporeal approach with tongue in groove repair.

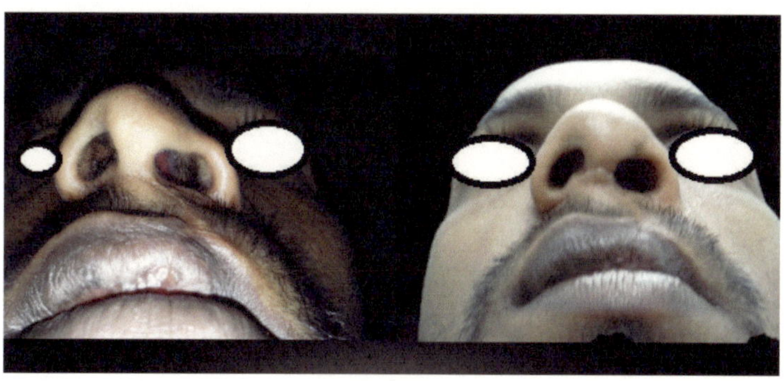

Figure 12.
Difficult 3: cleft nose.

With this approach one can attempt difficult cases as follows:

A happy surgeon-happy patient combination is one for which you should strive for (**Figures 9–12**).

Acknowledgements

Dr. A.V. Bhore, Director and Dr. K.J. Shinde, Prof. and Head of Department of ENT at SKN Medical College and Hospital for support and encouragement. Prof. Wolfgang Gubisch, Director, Department of Facial Plastic Surgery, Marien Hospital, Stuttgart, Germany for mentorship, inspiration and support for the study.

Conflict of interest

No conflict of interest.

Author details

Aditya Yeolekar
Smt. Kashibai Navale Medical College and General Hospital, Pune, India

*Address all correspondence to: adidoc@gmail.com

References

[1] Cook JA, Ramsay CR, Fayers P. Statistical analysis of learning curve effects in surgical trials. Clinical Trials. 2004;**1**(5):421-427

[2] Tang J, Tan S, Fang Q, Miao W, Tang A. Investigation of learning curve for cochlear implantation. Zhonghua Er Bi Yan Hou Tou Jing Wai Ke Za Zhi. 2014;**49**(8):649-653. DOI: 10.3760/cma.j.issn.1673-0860.2014.08.007

[3] Smith SJ, Erail G, Woon K, et al. Light at end of the tunnel. The learning curve associated with endoscopic trans sphenoidal skull base surgery. Skull Base. 2010;**20**(2):69-74. DOI: 10.1055/s-0029-1238214

[4] Liu CY, Yu EC, Lin SH, et al. Learning curve of septomeatoplasty. Auris Nasus Larynx. 2009;**36**(6):661-664. DOI: 10.1016/j.anl.2009.03.005. Epub 2009 May 2

[5] Luers JC, Damm M, Klussmann JP, et al. The learning curve of sialendoscopy with modular sial endoscopes. A single surgeons experience. Archives of Otolaryngology—Head & Neck Surgery. 2010;**136**(8):762-765. DOI: 10.1001/archoto.2010.109. Epub 2010 Jun 21

[6] Lohius PJFM. Advanced Caucasian and Mediterranean Rhinoplasty. Kugler Publications, 24-Apr-2014 p. 6. Chapter 1

[7] Daniel RK. Mastering Rhinoplasty. Springer-Verlag Berlin Heidelberg; 2010. ISBN 978-3-642-01401-7. eISBN 978-3-642-01402-4. DOI: 10.1007/978-3-642-01402-4

Section 3

Surgical Tips and Highlights

Chapter 3

Alar Rim Grafts

Pedro S. Arquero, Wenceslao M. Calonge, Daniel P. Espinoza and Diana Oesch

Abstract

Alar rim grafts date back to the 1950s for the correction of alar base in cleft lip nose. Cartilage struts under the anterior half of the *alae* of a pinched nose tip were popularised and the cartilage of the auricular concha became the donor site of choice for nasal procedures. Recently, some surgeons pointed to its potential role in aesthetic cases and added some technical refinements. These grafts are used for open and closed rhinoplasties. They usually consist of a rod of septal or auricular cartilage that we lay as reinforcement inside a pocket along the alar margin. Indications include the following: congenital or traumatic asymmetry, dynamic alar collapse, alar flare, primary retraction or notching, secondary (surgical or traumatic) retraction and malposition of the lateral cartilages (upwards or downwards). Harvesting and implanting techniques as well as the possible drawbacks are discussed.

Keywords: graft, alar, nose, cartilage, rhinoplasty

1. Introduction

In spite of deep inspiration, nasal tip maintains its general shape through different mechanisms. Major mechanisms include *medialis* and *lateralis* cartilages, the fibrous union between both *crus medialis* to the caudal septum and the ligaments that bind the caudal aspect of the superior lateral cartilages to the cephalic aspect of the inferior lateral cartilages. Secondary mechanisms encompass the cartilaginous septal dorsum, interdomal ligaments, the membranous septum, the nasal spine, the adherence between skin soft tissues and alar cartilages as well as the lateral alar walls (**Figure 1**).

Normal alar contour is defined by well-defined alar margins and extension from the tip lobe to the alar lobe. The inferior lateral cartilages act as a dynamic spring that can resist small traumatisms, providing some elasticity to the nasal tip to prevent a collapse of the nasal *alae* during inspiration.

Positioning of the alar cartilages is a fundamental element when planning a rhinoplasty. An overenthusiastic resection may cause their weakness and inability to perform their sustaining role.

An inadequate positioning of the alar cartilages entails an instable Anderson tripod with alar pinching. This may be a consequence of the resection of ligaments and the septal angle in order to achieve a reduction in nasal tip projection in open rhinoplasty procedures.

Less frequently, inborn asymmetries of the alar cartilages produce unbalance and rotation of the nasal tip. Moreover, some patients may suffer from a cephalad

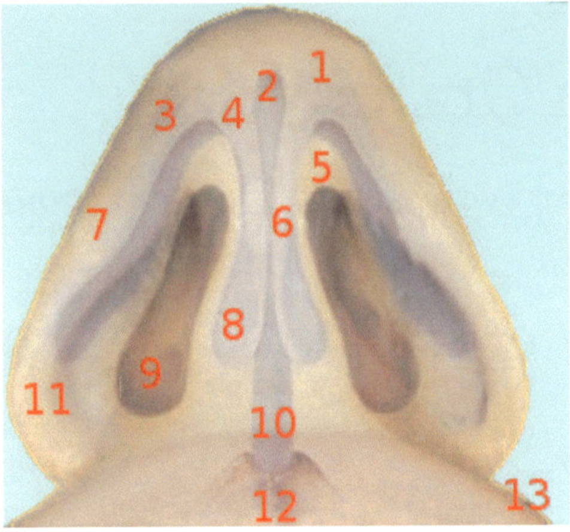

Figure 1.
A representation of the main cartilages from a basal perspective: 1. domus; 2. septal angle; 3. crus lateralis; 4. crus intermedia; 5. soft triangle; 6. crus medialis; 7. rima alaris; 8. 'feet' of the crura medialis; 9. nostrils; 10. caudal septum; 11. lobe of the nasal ala; 12. anterior nasal spine; and 13. nasolabial ridge.

rotation of the alar cartilages; they may orientate their main axis toward the inner cantus without giving adequate support to the external valve.

2. Historical notes

Alar and perialar rim grafts are rods or little splints made of cartilage. They are placed under the caudal margin of alar cartilages. They may be applied for primary and secondary rhinoplasty. Alar rim grafts were heralded as early as the 1950s by Fomon [1, 2] and Denecke [3] for the correction of alar base in cleft lip nose. Composite paranasal grafts on the nasal mucosa (instead of *under*) were an

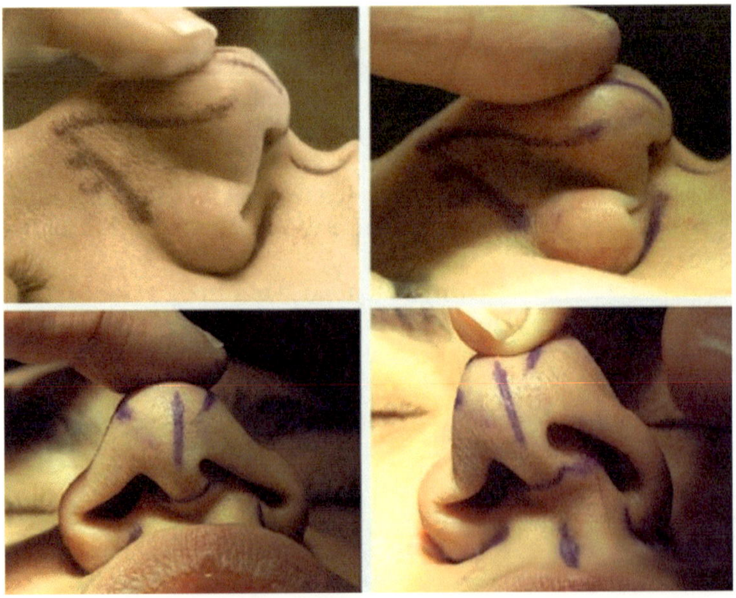

Figure 2.
Testing of the general elasticity and passive collapse of the nasal tip and alae.

Congenital asymmetry
Dynamic alar collapse
Alar flare (without functional impairment)
Primary retraction or notching
Secondary (surgical or traumatic) retraction as in pinched tip
Malposition of the lateral cartilages (upwards/downwards, bulbous tip, square tip)
Congenital microrrhinia (all nasal dimensions affected as seen in foetal alcoholic syndrome)

Table 1.
Main indications for alar rim grafts.

interesting, easier variation proposed by Farrior [4]. However, these techniques had a moderate predicament for the treatment of stenoses of the vestibule [5, 6]. In a parallel evolution, cartilage struts under the anterior half of the *alae* of a pinched nose tip were popularised, while the cartilage of the auricular concha became the donor site of choice for nasal procedures [7].

With greater emphasis focused on correcting the collapse of the internal valve, this approach by alar rim grafts was a sleeper. It was not until recent times when some surgeons [8–10] pointed to its potential role in aesthetic cases and added some technical refinements (**Figure 2**).

Alar rim grafts may be used for treatment and prevention of disorders of the nasal tip outline. They have been advised for the treatment of alar deformities. These deformities may stem not only from malposition or congenital hypoplasia of inferior lateral cartilages but also from a loss of continuity or a weakening of *crus lateralis* as a result of previous surgeries [11]. In rare cases, scar tissue may cause local *synechiae* that easily resolve with local section [12] (**Table 1**).

3. Pre-operative assessment

The position and dimension of the nasal *alae* must be assessed from frontal, lateral and basal points of view. As a rule of thumb, the distance between each inner cantus of the eyelids is roughly equivalent to the width of nasal base in frontal view. An ideal nasal base is schematised as an equilateral triangle. However, there is considerable interethnic variability. In shallow, general speaking, patients with East Asian and African ancestry may present a wider base [13]. The alar contour displays an oval nostril, and the alar fringe follows a smooth curvature with an inferior concavity. According to the distances between columella-nose axis and alar rim-nose axis, we may consider four different alterations of the alar position [14, 15] (**Figure 3A** and **B**):

- alar retraction—an elevation of the inferior concavity of the arch;
- hanging alar rim;
- retracted columella; and
- hanging columella—the inner mucosal lining of the medial aspect of each narine is conspicuous.

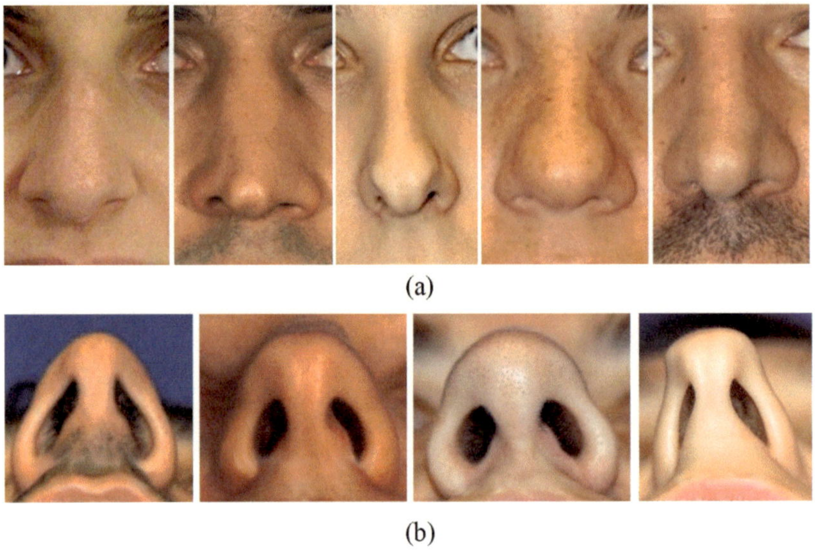

Figure 3.
(A) Anatomical variations and primary alterations of alar contour include (from left to right) pinched lobes, undulating alar cartilages, visible margins, bulbous tip and parallel orientation of both alar cartilages.
(B) Some features that may involve alar rim grafts as a treatment include (from left to right) lack of sustentation of alar rim, high positioned soft triangle, bulbous tip and square tip.

Functional primary disturbances may be the main motivation for a rhinoplasty (though they are also seen as an undesired side effect of a previous operation). These disturbances may cause difficulties in breathing, altered olfactory function, bleeding and frequent infection. Pre-operative rhinoscopy in order to exclude upper functional conditions (septal deviation, hypertrophic cornets, collapse of the upper internal valve and polyps) must be always carried out. A hanging tip is assessed by pinching the skin of the nasal dorsum. The collapse of the upper internal valve is sometimes evident after mild finger traction on the maxillary ascending apophysis. A cotton tip moisturised in adrenaline produces vasoconstriction and reduction in the size of hypertrophied cornets. A collapse of the lower valve may be corrected by gently opening the tweezers inside the air passage.

4. Surgical technique

Inspection of the nasal external valve constitutes an unavoidable step toward the end of any rhinoplasty procedure. Whenever we have performed a reduction of the projection of the nasal tip, we shall get an alar excess. Scar lines or excessive resection may entail a narrowing of the air passage. We use these grafts for open and closed rhinoplasties. The graft consists of a rod of septal or auricular cartilage (**Figure 4A, B** and **5**) that we lay as reinforcement inside a pocket along the alar margin. We perform an incision (less than 5 mm) on the hairy area of alar *vestibulum* (scarcely two-or-three millimetres away from the narine marge) by means of a number 11 blade. We use blunt scissors to create a double pocket backwards to the alar lobe and frontwards to the soft triangle (**Figure 6**). Some authors propose infiltration with 1% lidocaine with epinephrine in the skin caudal to the marginal incision [12]. In the so-created tunnels, we lay our rod of cartilage (from 1 × 6 mm up to 2 × 12 mm), from incision to back in the posterior tunnel and from incision to front in the anterior tunnel. We perform a single stitch in reabsorbable polydioxanone (PDS® 5/0). We must crush the anterior shaft with the tissue forceps in order

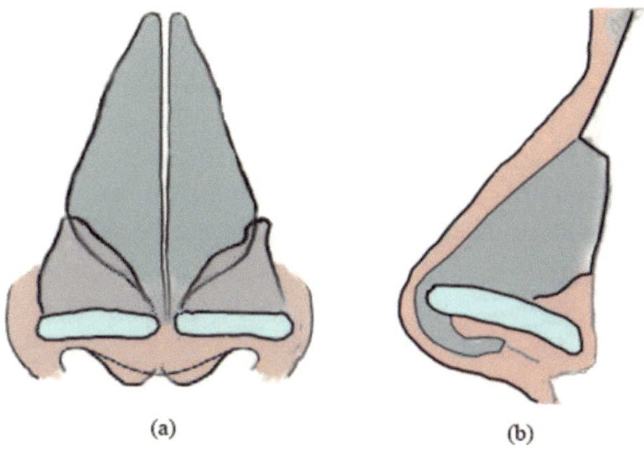

Figure 4.
(A) A sketch of the positioned alar rim graft in a frontal view. (B) The positioned alar rim graft in a lateral view.

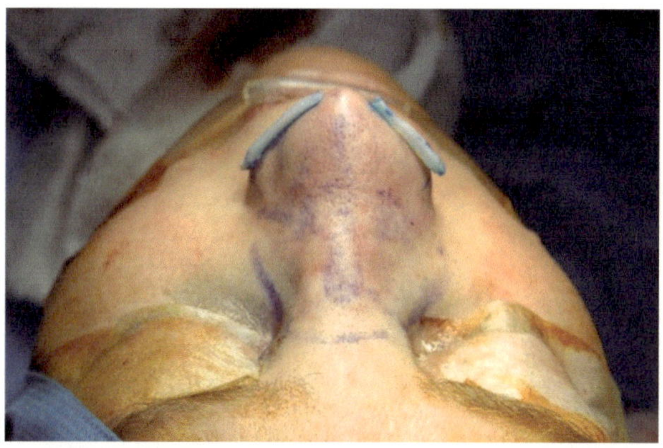

Figure 5.
Intraoperatory appreciation of the required length of grafts.

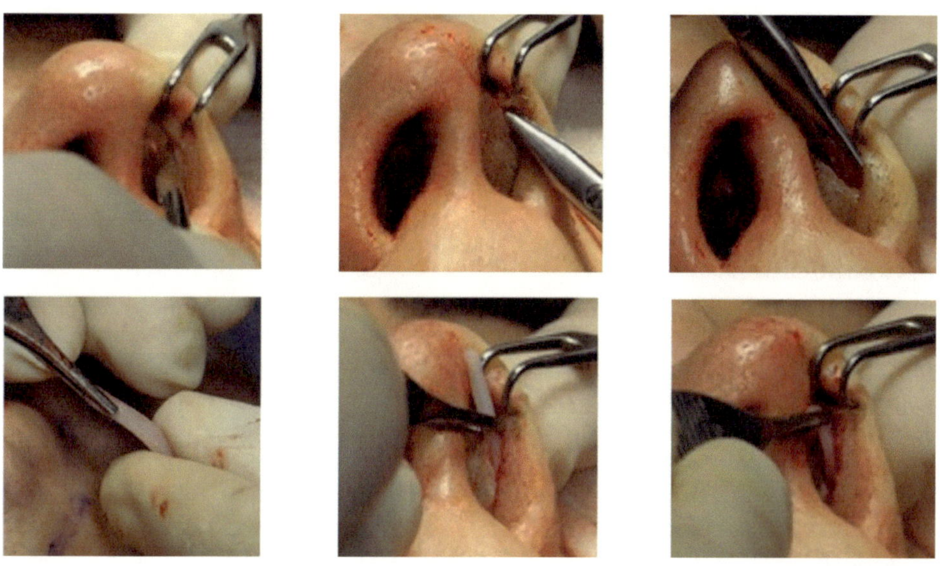

Figure 6.
Incision, blunt dissection and insertion of an alar rim graft.

to prevent it from exteriorizing through the skin. In any case, the graft should never extend anterior to the nasal tip [16, 17]. It must never widen the tip or be palpable [18]. We usually perform this step at the end of the procedure. We can check the final texture of the nasal tip and *alae* by pressing with fingertips or tissue forceps. Alar rim grafts allow us to caudally displace the alar rim margin up to 2 mm but this small gain reveals itself crucial in many cases. Whenever the alar rim graft is an isolated procedure, a safe, less traumatic way to incise the skin maybe achieved by using an ophthalmic slit blade [19].

5. Variations

When performing an open rhinoplasty, we use the same pre-rimal incision. Thus, we can check the symmetry of graft positioning. When performing a closed rhinoplasty, we place the grafts through a marginal incision (1 mm from the alar rim) and we extend the pocket frontwards to the soft triangle and backwards to the caudal end of the ala. We first lay the graft inside the posterior pocket and by careful sliding, we position its crushed edge inside the anterior pocket.

An alternative method involves conchal cartilage extension grafts fixed to the caudal margins of the lateral crura as described by Jang et al. [20]. This hybrid method focuses on correcting anterior contraction of the alar rim as seen in East Asian patients with nostril exposure. Alar vestibular skin is dissected at the end of an open approach for augmentation rhinoplasty. Conchal cartilage grafts are fashioned in a semilunar shape (13 mm × 6 mm) and sutured to the caudal margins of each *crus lateralis*.

Articulated alar rim grafts [21, 22] stand as an interesting concept. In this widespread variation, the anterior margin of each alar rim graft is sutured to the tip complex instead of just being freely sited in a pocket. Emphasis is mainly made to stabilise the nasal tip.

A peculiar variation [23] elevates a 2–3 mm flap from the caudal portion of the *crus lateralis*, pulls it caudally and extends it with a cartilage graft. This extension of the alar rim flap is placed along the alar rim for support.

Selected cases of external nasal valve collapse as an isolated condition have been treated by a microinvasive technique that creates the pocket from the cutaneous, facial aspect of the posterior margin of the ala [24].

Needless to say, versatile surgeons should bear in mind alternative donor sites as part of their armamentarium [25]. A posterior incision is the less conspicuous choice when taking conchal grafts Adequate semicompressive dressings and anaesthetic infiltration of the margins of the skin (for instance with bupivacaine or ropivacaine) would minimise haematoma and post-operative pain in this donor area.

6. Complications

As with any surgical procedures, patients should be informed about potential problems as transient inflammation, haemorrhage, haematoma, seroma, adherences, conspicuous scarring, keloids and pigmentation alterations. The same goes for undesirable infectious conditions as chondritis, osteitis, myositis and abscess. More specific conditions are paraesthesia, loss of temperature sensation and partial resorption of the cartilaginous graft. Jarring right-left asymmetry of the grafts may entail pyramid deviation.

Local necrosis and extrusion of the graft are very rarely seen. They may be the result of local traumatism or inadequate dressing as well as previous ischaemic features as seen in chain smoking (**Figures 7–10**).

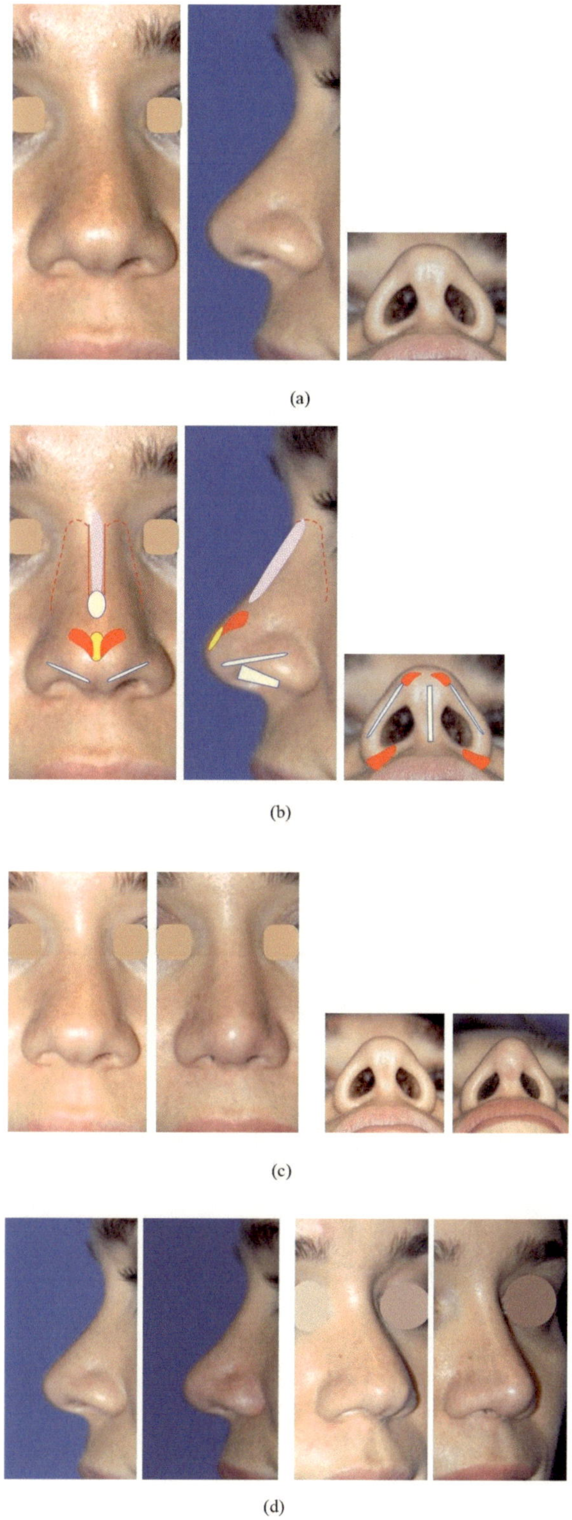

Figure 7.
(A) Broad, bilobed nasal tip in a 27-year-old female patient. Slight deviation of dorsum and retracted columella. (B) Surgical planning for the patient in ***Figure 5A****. This patient underwent lipectomy (yellow), cephalic resection of alar cartilages (red), caudal extension graft (from septum), submucous section of triangle area, medial and lateral fracture (spiked line), septal cartilage graft over tip region, septal cartilage graft inside alar rim. (C) and (D) Post-operative result of patient in (A).*

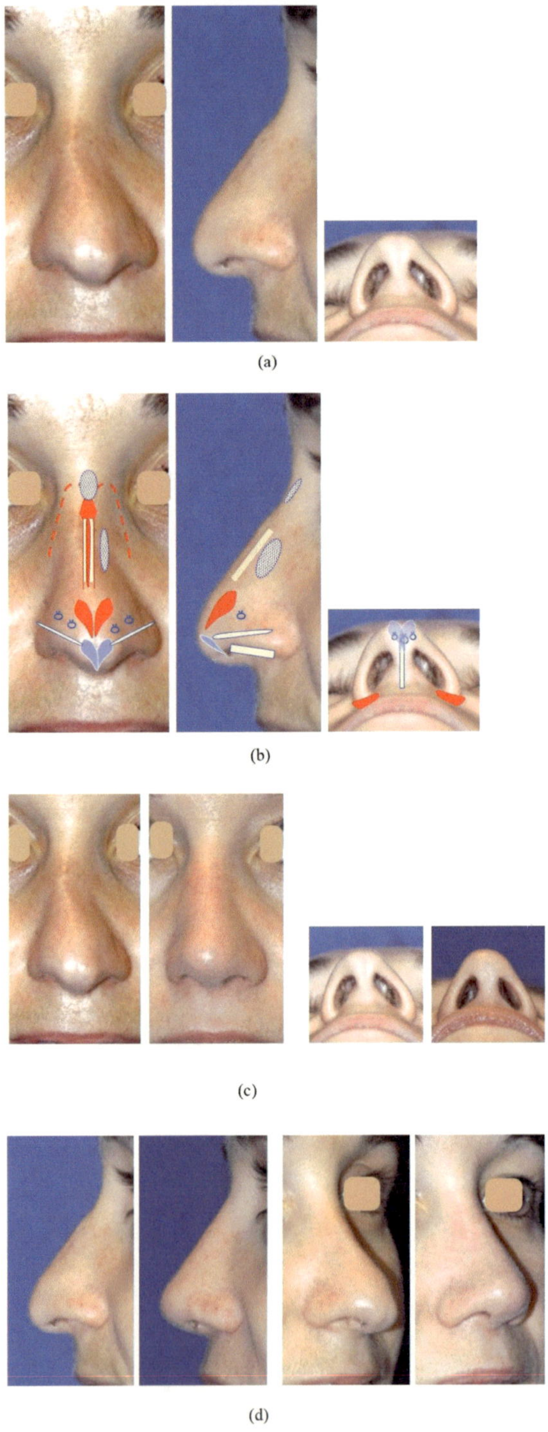

Figure 8.
(A) A 32-year-old female patient suffering for traumatic deviation. Hanging tip, acute nasolabial angle, broad tip and unbalance between lobe and alae. (B) Surgical planning for the patient in ***Figure 6A****. A trans-columellar incision was extended along pre-rimal areas. The procedure included a partial septoplasty (red), tension-discharging incisions on the left side, dorsal expansion grafts, a columellar stick graft, cephalic resection of alar cartilages, several interdomal, intradomal and intraalar stitches, as well as septal cartilage graft to the left cartilaginous wall, a suspension-rotation suture of the crus medialis, predomal grafts (light blue), a medial and lateral fracture (interrupted line), a batten graft to the radix, pre-rimal grafts and a resection with rotation of the skin and mucosa of the alae. (C) and (D) Comparison between pre-operative and post-operative result of patient in (A).*

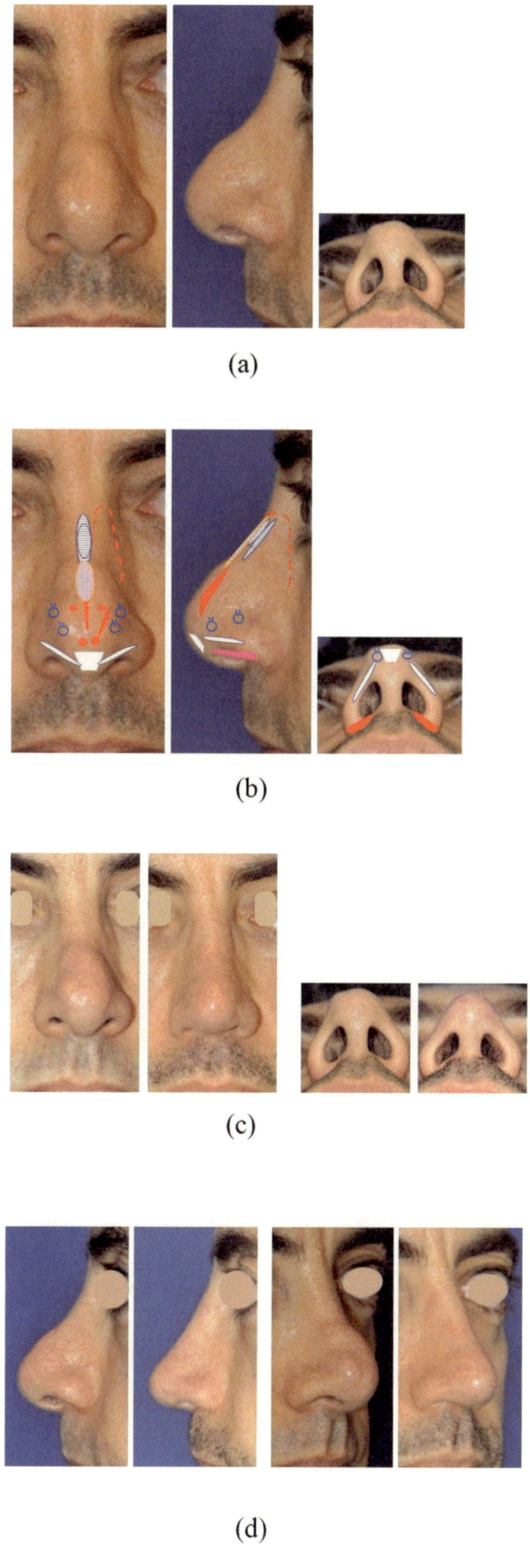

Figure 9.
(A) A 35-year-old male patient with supratip deformation after secondary rhinoplasty. He showed a thick skin, a saddle (broad and flat) dorsum as well as an asymmetric, pinched tip, other features include an osseous dehiscence on the left side and malpositioned, undulating alae. (B) Surgical planning for patient in (A). (C) and (D) Comparison between pre-operative and post-operative result of patient in (A).

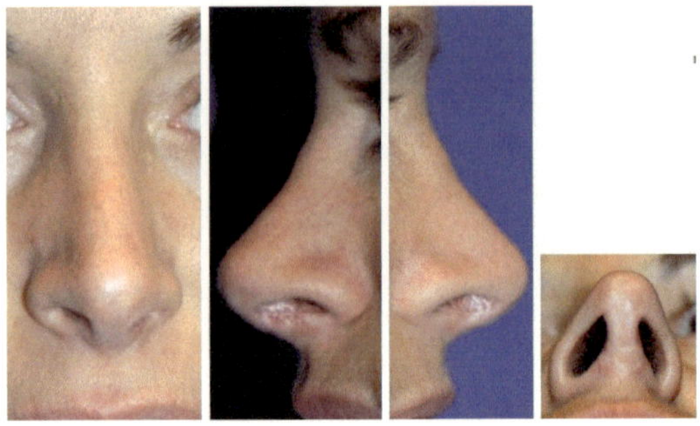

(a)

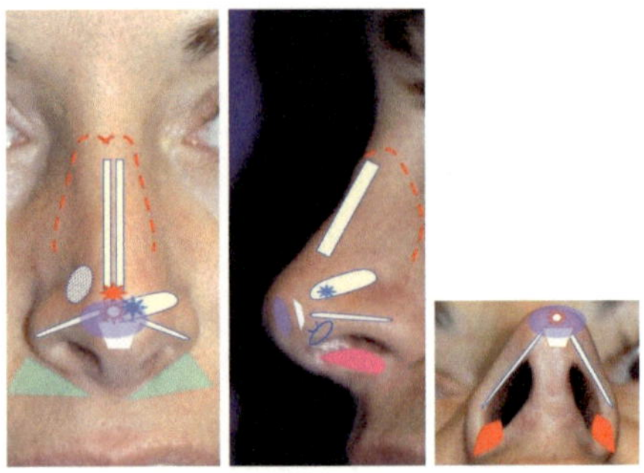

(b)

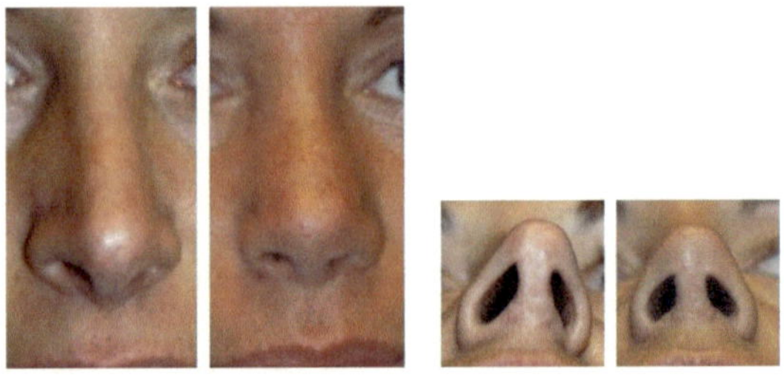

(c)

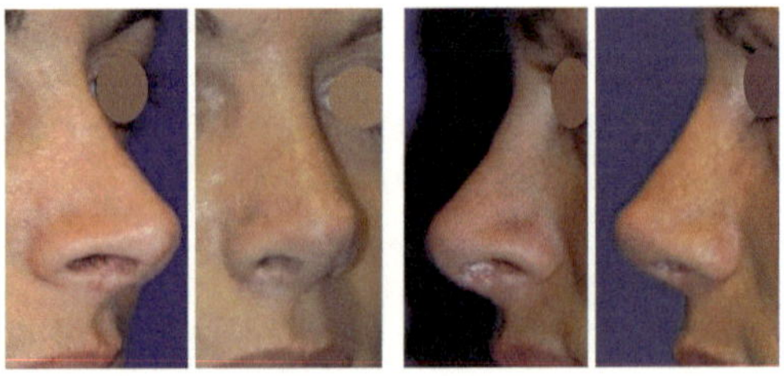

(d)

Figure 10.
(A) Secondary rhinoplasty in a 29-year-old female patient that showed deviation, irregularities of her dorsum, upper valve collapse, pinched tip, light alar retraction, hanging columella and maxillary hypotrophy. (B) Surgical planning for the patient in **Figure 8A** *included an osteocartilaginous septoplasty with removal of previous graft and fibrotic tissue (red star). The procedure involved reconstruction of the left alar cartilage (blue star), expansor grafts for dorsum, batten alar graft on the right lateral wall, a left alar graft, a predomal graft, a fixation suture between crus medialis and caudal septum, pre-rimal grafts, a lateral fracture (spiked line), partial resection of the mucosa of the membranous septum, an expansion mesh of polypropylene on the maxilla and partial resection of the skin and mucosa of the alae. (C) and (D) Comparison between pre-operative and post-operative result of patient in (A).*

7. Conclusion

These grafts are useful to prevent an alar retraction and post-operative shifts on those patients that show primary alterations of alar outline. They provide support and steadiness for the alar rim by creating a structure that counteracts the forces of scar contraction [26–29]. Whenever we use them we shall prevent descent (or rotation) of caudal margin of alar cartilages and a trilobulate, pinched nose. At the same time, we enhance a correct functioning of the external valve and prevent its collapse.

These grafts are also very useful for the treatment of pinched, nasal tips with a very long *crus intermedium*, i.e. lack of sustentation of skin in the soft triangle. We may use them as a complement for domal sutures and alar grafts in order to compensate the modifications that these procedures induce on the sustaining tip structures; they favour projection and balance of the nasal tip while preserving the function of external valve. They allow us to provide triangularity to the nasal base, by re-establishing the Anderson tripod, as well as to preserve the pyramidal shape of nasal tip. This will help to achieve a natural allure of the nasal tip contour.

Author details

Pedro S. Arquero[1†], Wenceslao M. Calonge[2*†], Daniel P. Espinoza[3] and Diana Oesch[2]

1 Clinica Arquero, Madrid, Spain

2 Clinique de Genolier, Genolier, Switzerland

3 Centre Feel Well, Geneva, Switzerland

*Address all correspondence to: wcalonge@yahoo.es

† These authors equally contributed to the work.

References

[1] Fomon S, Bell JW, Berger EL, Goldman IB, Neivert H, Schattner A. Management of deformities of lower cartilaginous vault. A.M.A. Archives of Otolaryngology. 1951;**54**(5):467-472

[2] Fomon S, Bell JW, Lubart J, Schattner A, Syracuse VR. Rhinoplastic problems in the lower cartilaginous vault. Archives of Otolaryngology. 1964;**79**:512-521

[3] Denecke HJ, Meyer R. Plastische Operationen an Kopf und Hals. In: Korrigierende und Rekonstruktive Nasenplastik. Berlin: Springer; 1964

[4] Farrior RT. The problem of the unilateral cleft lip nose. A composite operation for revisión of the secondary deformity. Laryngoscope. 1962;**72**:289-352

[5] Janeke JB, Wright WK. Studies on the support of the nasal tip. Archives of Otolaryngology. 1971;**93**(5):458-464

[6] Vecchione TR. Reconstruction of the ala and nostril sill using proximal composite grafts. Annals of Plastic Surgery. 1980;**5**(2):148-150

[7] Orticoechea M. A new method for total reconstruction of the nose: The ears as donor areas. Clinics in Plastic Surgery. 1981;**8**(3):481-505

[8] Troell RJ, Powell N, Riley RW, Li KK. Evaluation of a new procedure for nasal alar rim and valve collapse: Nasal alar rim reconstruction. Otolaryngology and Head and Neck Surgery. 2000;**122**(2):204-211

[9] Rohrich RJ, Raniere J Jr, Ha RY. The alar contour graft: Correction and prevention of alar rim deformities in rhinoplasty. Plastic and Reconstructive Surgery. 2002;**109**(7):2495-2505

[10] Toriumi DM, Checcone MA. New concepts in nasal tip contouring. Facial Plastic Surgery Clinics of North America. 2009;**17**(1):55-90

[11] Daniel RK, Palhazi P, Gerbault O, Kosins AM. Rhinoplasty: The lateral crura-alar ring. Aesthetic Surgery Journal. 2014;**34**(4):526-537

[12] Alexander AJ, Shah AR, Constantinides MS. Alar retraction: Etiology, treatment, and prevention. JAMA Facial Plastic Surgery. 2013;**15**(4):268-274

[13] Tas S, Colakoglu S, Lee BT. Nasal base retraction: A treatment algorithm. Aesthetic Surgery Journal. 2017;**37**(6):640-653

[14] Ellenbogen R, Bazell G. Nostrilplasty: Raising, lowering, widening, and symmetry correction of the alar rim. Aesthetic Surgery Journal. 2002;**22**(3):227-237

[15] Unger JG, Roostaeian J, Small KH, Pezeshk RA, Lee MR, Harris R, et al. Alar contour grafts in rhinoplasty: A safe and reproducible way to refine alar contour aesthetics. Plastic and Reconstructive Surgery. 2016;**137**(1):52-61

[16] Gruber RP, Fox P, Peled A, Belek KA. Grafting the alar rim: Application as anatomical graft. Plastic and Reconstructive Surgery. 2014;**134**(6):880e-887e

[17] Toriumi DM, Josen J, Weinberger M, Tardy ME Jr. Use of alar batten grafts for correction of nasal valve collapse. Archives of Otolaryngology—Head & Neck Surgery. 1997;**123**:802-808

[18] Guyuron B, Bigdeli Y, Sajjadian A. Dynamics of the alar rim graft. Plastic and Reconstructive Surgery. 2015;**135**(4):981-986

[19] Li YK, Greensmith A. Facilitated alar rim graft placement with an

ophthalmic slit blade. Plastic and Reconstructive Surgery. Global Open. 2018;**6**(4):e1721

[20] Jang YJ, Kim SM, Lew DH, Song SY. Simple correction of alar retraction by conchal cartilage extension grafts. Archives of Plastic Surgery. 2016;**43**(6):564-569 [Epub Nov 18, 2016]

[21] Goodrich JL, Wong BJ. Optimizing the soft tissue triangle, alar margin furrow, and alar ridge aesthetics: Analysis and use of the articulate alar rim graft. Facial Plastic Surgery. 2016;**32**(6):646-655

[22] Ballin AC, Kim H, Chance E, Davis RE. The articulated alar rim graft: Reengineering the conventional alar rim graft for improved contour and support. Facial Plastic Surgery. 2016;**32**(4):384-397

[23] Kemaloğlu CA, Altıparmak M. The alar rim flap: A novel technique to manage malpositioned lateral crura. Aesthetic Surgery Journal. 2015;**35**(8):920-926

[24] Deroee AF, Younes AA, Friedman O. External nasal valve collapse repair: The limited alar-facial stab approach. The Laryngoscope. 2011;**121**(3):474-479

[25] Field LM. Nasal alar rim reconstruction utilizing the crus of the helix, with several alternatives for donor site closure. The Journal of Dermatologic Surgery and Oncology. 1986;**12**(3):253-258

[26] Losquadro WD, Bared A, Toriumi DM. Correction of the retracted alar base. Facial Plastic Surgery. 2012;**28**(2):218-224

[27] Boahene KD, Hilger PA. Alar rim grafting in rhinoplasty: Indications, technique, and outcomes. Archives of Facial Plastic Surgery. 2009;**11**(5):285-289

[28] Kalan A, Kenyon GS, Seemungal TA. Treatment of external nasal valve (alar rim) collapse with an alar strut. The Journal of Laryngology and Otology. 2001;**115**(10):788-791

[29] Cárdenas-Camarena L, Guerrero MT. Use of cartilaginous autografts in nasal surgery: 8 years of experience. Plastic and Reconstructive Surgery. 1999;**103**(3):1003-1014

Chapter 4

Saddle Nose: A Systematic Approach

Marianetti Tito Matteo

Abstract

The saddle nose deformity is always associated to cartilaginous or bone defects. It could have congenital, traumatic, infectious or iatrogenic origin. Its correction consists not only in a camouflage, but also it is important to reconstruct the missing structure. In this chapter, we will discuss about all aspect of the saddle nose and we will propose a different therapeutical approach (septum, concha or costal grafts) in relation to the severity of the defects (with a personal classification). The classification is also based on the presence or absence of the nasal septum, which is a fundamental aspect that we must take into account when approaching nasal reconstruction. We will discuss the technical aspect of the rib graft harvesting and its use to reconstruct the nasal structure.

Keywords: saddle nose, rib graft, nasal reconstruction

1. Introduction

Saddle nose is a pathological deformity characterized by loss of nasal dorsal height due to osseocartilaginous collapse.

While the cause can be congenital, for example, syphilis or intrauterine trauma, most cases are due to trauma of the nasal septum and pyramid, Wegener granulomatosis, relapsing polychondritis, cocaine abuse, and previous rhinoplasty. The removal of an excessive amount of the bone and/or cartilage during a prior operation is the most frequent cause.

Saddle nose is one of the most difficult morpho-functional deformities of the nose to correct, as it entails not only masking with a graft but also planned anatomical reconstruction of all the structures involved. Grafts obtained from septal or conchal cartilage, sutured in overlapping layers so as to increase the thickness where necessary, can be sufficient in cases of low to medium severity. The presence of septal remnants can be exploited to combine septal grafts with grafts of auricular concha in order to increase the thickness of the final graft. There is instead less agreement on the choice of material for use in reconstruction in cases of greater severity, where the absence of cartilage is often combined with the absence of the bony support of the nasal pyramid. The ideal graft material must be nontoxic, non-carcinogenic, non-allergenic, nondestructive with respect to adjacent tissues, non-resorbable, readily available, and sterilizable as well as easy to shape and to remove if necessary.

The variety of autogenous (bony and cartilaginous), homologous (irradiated cartilage), and alloplastic grafts put forward in the literature attests to the

IntechOpen

nonexistence of one "ideal" material. Alloplastic grafts have a tendency toward extrusion and infection, and homologous grafts are characterized by the highest rate of resorption. The bone is difficult to shape, requires solid stabilization, and can be reabsorbed. In the end, despite its tendency toward distortion, costal cartilage remains at present the material of choice for the correction of severe cases of saddle nose.

It should also be pointed out, on the basis of the majority of cases presented in the literature, that cartilaginous grafts give rise to the fewest problems as regards shaping, attachment, and infection. The only negative data regarding resorption is, however, limited in the case of autologous cartilage and generally ceases in the first few months after the operation.

1.1 Autologous grafts

1.1.1 Bone

The bone is the material most commonly employed to remedy saddle nose over the last century. The first to use the autologous bone for nasal reconstruction was Ollier in 1861, who inserted a piece of the frontal bone in an Indian flap. The material is mostly taken from the cranium and the iliac crest [1, 2]. The bone cannot be regarded as a material of choice, however, because it tends to be reabsorbed when inserted into the nasal dorsum. Complications at the donor site and the fact that grafts of this nature create a dorsum of excessive rigidity are further reasons why the use of autologous bone in cases of saddle nose has been practically abandoned today [3].

1.1.2 Cartilage

Currently regarded as the graft material closest to the ideal, autologous cartilage presents the following characteristics: (1) it causes little reaction in the tissues of the recipient site; (2) it possesses the combination of rigidity, elasticity, and flexibility required to reconstruct the contours of the nose; (3) it can resist the traction forces of wound healing; (4) it can survive without functional use (unlike the bone); (5) it is available in large amounts; and (6) it is easy to reshape and survives over time without the perichondrium. Tardy reports no cases of infection or rejection in 6000 cartilaginous grafts. It has also been shown that resorption is short-lived and limited to the initial postoperative period [2, 4].

In cases of low or moderate severity, cartilage from the nasal septum or auricular concha can be used. In more severe cases, a graft of costal cartilage constitutes the preferred therapeutic option. This cartilage is hyaline and proves to be rigid and fragile (**Figure 1**). Always available in large amounts and thicknesses, it is sufficiently rigid for use in cases where it is necessary to counter the retraction of thick, inelastic, cicatricial tissues. While the material is usually harvested from the ninth and tenth ribs, the sixth, seventh, and eighth are preferable in the case of female patients, as the incision is thus made in the inframammary fold and the postoperative scar is not visible. Gunter et al. [5] suggest that a CT scan of the sternal-costal region should be carried out in the case of adult patients to ascertain the degree of calcification of the cartilaginous portion of the ribs.

The incision (about 5 cm) must be performed horizontally in the medial (cartilaginous) portion of the rib. In harvesting material from the sixth, seventh, and eighth ribs, it must be borne in mind that their medial portion is covered by the rectus abdominis muscle of the abdomen (**Figure 2**). The fascia of this muscle must be cut and the fibers opened out in the same direction as the fascicle. The ninth and

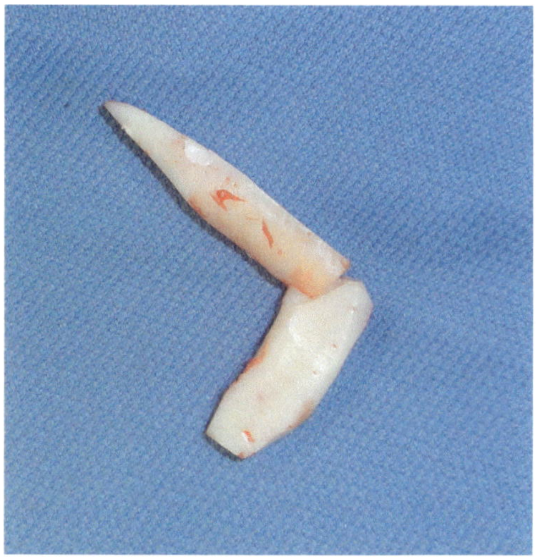

Figure 1.
Costal cartilage used to reconstruct the "L-structure" of the septum.

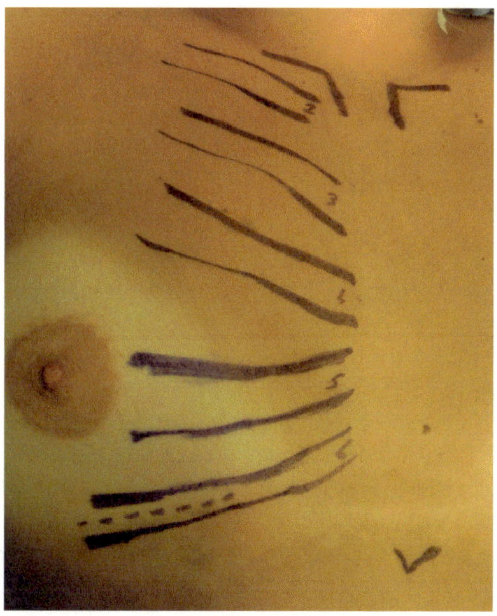

Figure 2.
Preoperative drawing of the second to sixth rib of a patient.

tenth ribs are instead located at the side of the rectus abdominis muscle. Once the outer surface of the rib has been exposed, it must be separated from the intercostal muscles, which can be facilitated on the inner side by the use of a specific curved rib elevator (**Figure 3**).

The perichondrium can be separated from the rib for subsequent use to cover any residual irregularities of the nasal dorsum.

Particular care must be taken in detaching the inferior portion of the rib, as this is where the anterior intercostal branches of the internal thoracic (or mammary) artery, the venae comitantes, and the intercostal nerves are all situated. It is important to identify the joint of the bony and cartilaginous portions so as to harvest the largest possible amount of cartilage. Once the portion of the rib required has been

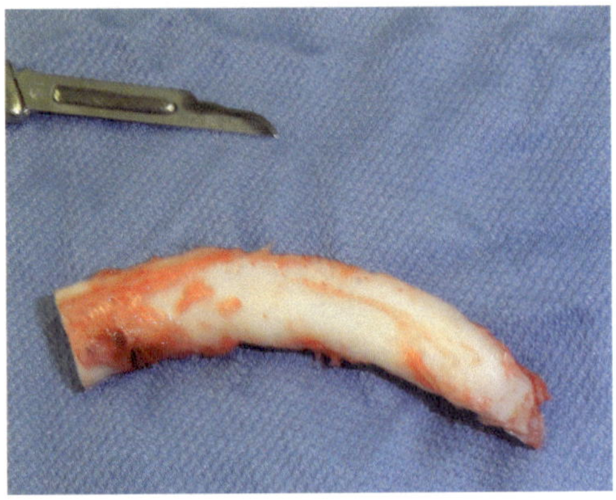

Figure 3.
Harvesting of the cartilaginous segment of the sixth rib.

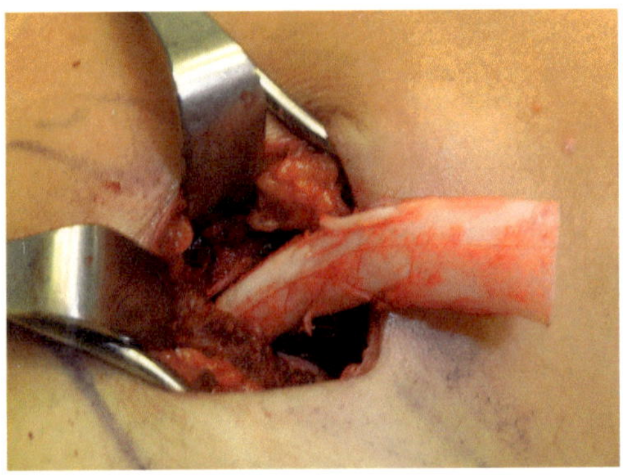

Figure 4.
Intraoperative view of the costal harvesting.

exposed and detached, it can be removed by excision, using a scalpel with sturdy blade; after which it is necessary to make sure that the pleura below is undamaged. The cavity thus left is filled with a saline solution, and the anesthetist is asked to increase the pressure in the airways, making sure that no bubbles appear in the cavity.

A considerable amount of cartilage can be obtained from the rib, and more than one can be harvested with no postoperative functional deficit (**Figure 4**).

It is very important to suture the remaining perichondrium tightly so as to seal off the empty space left after harvesting the rib.

The major problem of costal cartilage is its tendency to become distorted [6]. Various methods have been put forward for the prevention of this complication. Gibson and Davis [7] demonstrated that "balanced cross-sectional carving" (removal of the perichondrium and a strip of cartilage from the outer and inner sides with respect to the thorax and the use of the cartilage in the middle) reduced the tendency toward distortion considerably. Gibson then stated, however, in a later publication that distortion of the cartilage could only be prevented by not harvesting it. Some authors investigated the molecular basis of the tendency toward distortion of the cartilage and showed that certain protein-polysaccharide complexes inhibits the intracartilaginous stress causing distortion, an interesting discovery that has, however, had no clinical application [8]. Gunter et al. [9] have demonstrated that distortion of the harvested costal cartilage is significantly reduced by the insertion of a Kirschner thread. While the different authors all agree that the distortion peaks 15–30 minutes after harvesting, some claim that it exists only in the first half of an hour and others claim that it can take place even months after the operation. The most superficial and deepest layers of the costal cartilage harvested are those that undergo the greatest distortion according to the rule of cross-sectional carving. Common experience suggests that this is accelerated if the cartilage is immersed in a saline solution immediately after removal.

Complications in the area of the donor site are very infrequent. They can include pneumothorax, localized postoperative atelectasis, and unsightly scarring. Postoperative pain is instead common and can be prevented or reduced by injecting local anesthetic into the subperichondrial space before the final suturing [10–11].

1.2 Alloplastic grafts

While alloplastic grafts present a high risk of infection and extrusion, many surgeons make use of them at first because they are readily available and, above all, avoid any complications at the donor site. Prostheses of silicone (Silastic) are still widely used by many authors to reconstruct the dorsum in cases of saddle nose, probably because they prove to be easy to handle and to remove in the event of infection [12–15]. Milward reports extrusion rates of up to 55%, however, and Deva et al. complications in 9.7% of cases [12, 13]. Other materials used include polytetrafluoroethylene and hydroxyapatite. Complications have been reported in 2.6–5% of cases for Gore-Tex and 5% for hydroxyapatite [16, 17].

Another synthetic material frequently used at present with an apparently lower percentage of complications is porous high-density polyethylene (PHDPE: MEDPOR surgical implants, Porex Surgical), which has been employed in cranio-maxillofacial surgery for 20 years now and is of proven tolerability. This porous alloplastic material (pores of about 150 microns in diameter) is not degradable in vivo and permits the fibrointegration of soft tissues. Once this has taken place, it proves to be stable, and the risk of extrusion and infection diminishes over the years. Romo et al. suggest covering the MEDPOR graft with a homologous graft of purified acellular human derma in order to taper the edges and make the dorsum less rigid and more natural in appearance. Even though this is one of the alloplastic materials most frequently used at present, Romo reports complications in 3–4% of cases [17].

1.3 Classification and therapeutic algorithm

Tardy's classification of saddle nose has three increasing degrees of severity: minimum, moderate, and major [2]. The first degree involves slight accentuation of the depression of the supratip, 1–2 millimeters above the ideal. The presence can be observed in such cases of a dorsal "pseudo-hump" in the upper third of the nasal pyramid caused by collapse of the other two thirds. If saddle nose deformity is due to the absence of the caudal septum, there will also be a certain degree of columellar retraction. Saddle nose of moderate and major severity presents greater depression of the dorsum due to the loss of osseocartilaginous support.

The classification of Daniel and Brenner [18] instead distinguishes six types of saddle nose:

(1) Type 0 (pseudo-saddle nose) comprises patients who present depression of the cartilaginous dorsum due to prior rhinoplasty. (2) Type I (minor) includes cases with excessive depression of the supratip and columellar retraction caused by weakening of the cartilaginous septum. (3) Type II (moderate) is characterized by collapse of the cartilaginous ridge, columellar retraction, and loss of support for the tip. (4) Type III (major) comprises more severe cases with the total absence of support for the cartilaginous ridge, the columella, and the nasal tip. (5) Type IV

(severe) involves the total absence of osseocartilaginous support, often combined with septal perforation, depression of the osseocartilaginous dorsum, columellar retraction, and the loss of tip projection. (6) Type V (catastrophic) comprises cases that require local or free flaps for reconstruction and are often combined with deformity of other neighboring regions of the face. The authors correlate each of the different types with a therapeutic approach, increasing in complexity in relation to the tissue deficit involved, and a specific etiology.

It is, however, often difficult in practical terms to identify a particular case of saddle nose as belonging to one category or another of an overly specific classification characterized by common etiologies, clinical characteristics, and therapeutic approaches. As Murakami says, "variability exists to large extent, because the saddle nose deformity is not a single entity but rather a spectrum of abnormalities."

On the other hand, the practical need is felt for quick classification of saddle nose as a prerequisite for deciding how to correct it.

The original classification put forward here as a more practical tool involves three degrees of severity and takes the presence or absence of the nasal septum as the primary factor in determining the surgical treatment required.

Degree I (slight): depression <2 mm with respect to the ideal height of the dorsum: septum present (**Figure 5a**).

Degree II (moderate): depression of 2–5 mm with respect to the ideal height of the dorsum:

(a) cartilaginous septum present or partially present (**Figure 6a**) and
(b) septum absent (**Figure 7a**)

Degree III (severe): depression >5 mm with respect to the ideal height of the dorsum: septum absent (**Figure 8a**).

The resulting therapeutic algorithm is as follows:

I: Onlay grafts from the nasal septum (**Figure 5b**).
IIa: Onlay grafts from the nasal septum and/or auricular concha (**Figure 6b**).
IIb: Reconstruction of the septum and dorsum with auricular concha (**Figure 7b**).
III: Reconstruction of the septum and dorsum with costal cartilage (**Figure 8b**).

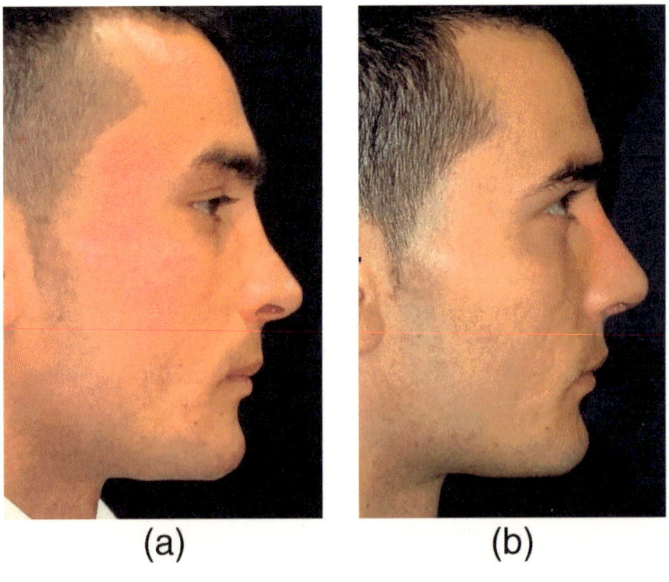

Figure 5.
(a) Preoperative view of a patient affected by saddle nose deformity degree I (slight). (b) Postoperative profile view of the same patient of (a).

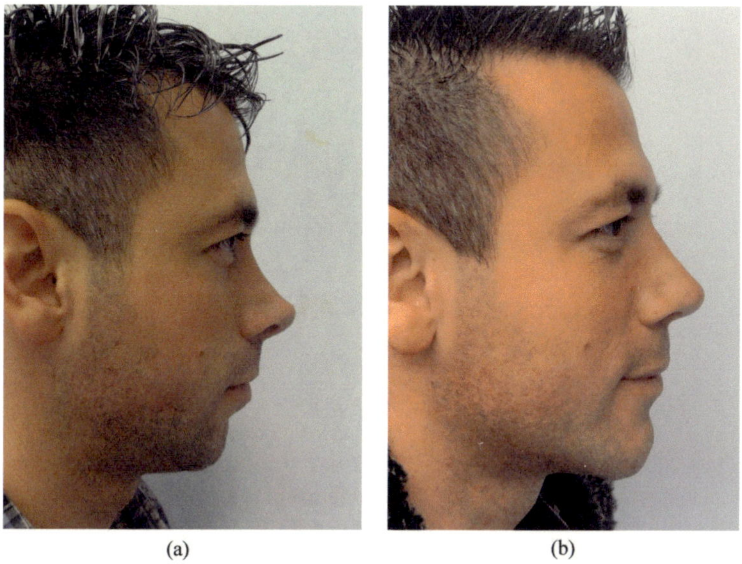

Figure 6.
(a) Preoperative view of a patient affected by saddle nose deformity degree IIa (moderate with cartilaginous septum present). (b) Postoperative profile view of the same patient of (a).

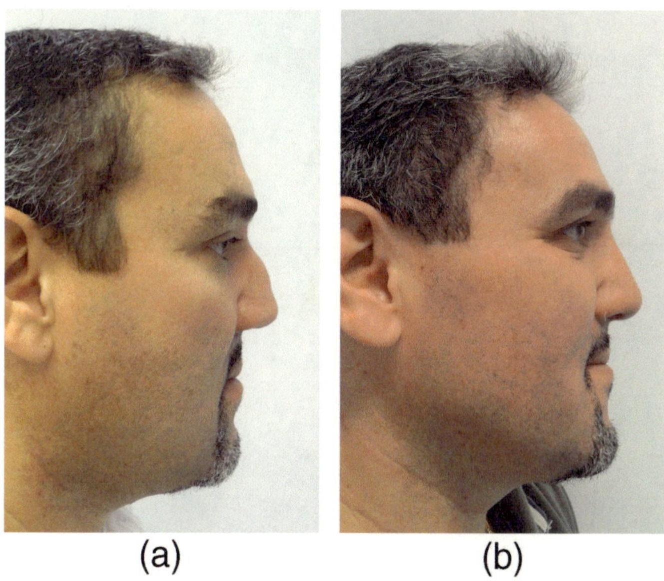

Figure 7.
(a) Preoperative view of a patient affected by saddle nose deformity degree IIb (moderate with cartilaginous septum absent). (b). Postoperative profile view of the same patient of (a).

The ideal height of the dorsum differs for men and women, coinciding in the first case with the line from the nasion to the tip-defining points (with suitable projection of the tip) and positioned about 2 mm caudally from the same in the second.

The presence or absence of the nasal septum, as ascertained clinically not only by palpation and anterior rhinoscopy but also by radiological means like RMN for greater accuracy, is of crucial importance in deciding how to correct the deformity (**Figure 9**).

The primary objective must be to restore support for the nose and then to obtain the desired appearance. The reconstruction can be thus described as composite with a bottom layer of support and an upper layer of esthetic importance. In cases I and

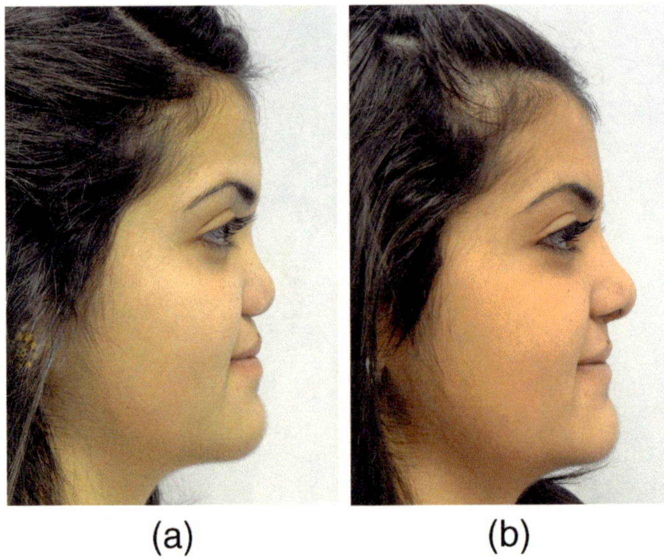

Figure 8.
(a) Preoperative view of a patient affected by saddle nose deformity degree III (severe). (b). Postoperative profile view of the same patient of (a).

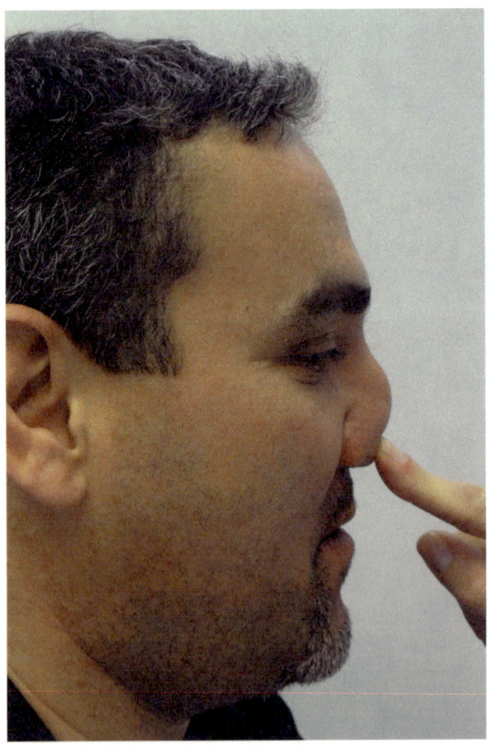

Figure 9.
Clinical sign of absent septal support.

IIa, where the septum is present and support exists, onlay grafts can be used to correct the deformity. The material can be taken from the present or residual septum and from the cartilage of the auricular concha if this proves insufficient.

The onlay graft must be carefully shaped to make sure that it is not perceptible to sight or touch after the operation. To this end, incisions can be made halfway through the thickness of the cartilage in order to obtain a more or less curved shape as required. The cartilage can be given as inverted V, inverted U, or A shape by means of greenwood fractures.

It must also be oval, wider in the middle, and narrower at the top and bottom, in order to follow the natural shape of the dorsum.

An inverted V graft offers superior adaptation and stability than a flat one. As it consists of a single layer, it can only be used for patients requiring a minimal increase in the dorsum. If more is needed, a pillar of cartilage can be sutured beneath the inverted V so as to create a solid A-shaped structure. This stabilizing pillar can be secured closer to or farther from the top of the inverted V in order to vary the degree of gap between the arms of the V and increase or decrease the height of the graft. Both the inverted V and the A shape present, however, a very acute angle at the top, which can make the dorsum look too narrow in patients with very thin skin. In such cases, it proves useful to make further incisions halfway through the thickness on either side of the median incision so as to obtain an inverted U shape, which is closer to the natural curvature of the nasal dorsum and proves more stable on insertion into the same. Even in cases when only a localized dorsal defect is present, it is usually preferable, where possible, to use a graft covering the area from the nasion to the septal angle in order to reduce the irregularities, obtain the best esthetic result, and reduce the possibility of the graft being moved out of position. In order to secure the onlay graft, a very precise pouch must be created cephalically so as to prevent movement out of position. Caudally, it is instead possible to secure the graft to the septum or the alar cartilages, suturing in this case being obviously facilitated by the open approach. In order to obtain greater stability, a median incision of about 5 mm can be made in the caudal edge of the graft so as to obtain two small strips of cartilage for suturing to the lateral crura.

Some authors advise securing the graft also cephalically by means of transcutaneous sutures to be removed after 7–10 days. One further tip when using onlay grafts is to taper the edges carefully in order to prevent the creation of "steps" perceptible to sight or touch after the operation.

Degree IIb involves moderate depression of the nasal dorsum and the absence of septal support. In such cases, while costal cartilage is a possibility, reconstruction of the L-shaped structure of caudal dorsal support with auricular cartilage is unquestionably preferable given the almost total absence of undesirable esthetic-functional consequences. It is in any case generally preferable, whenever possible, to harvest material from the auricular concha rather than the rib, not least in terms of acceptability to the patient. Even though its elasticity and natural curvature do not make conchal cartilage an ideal material for reconstruction of the nasal septum, it is possible to obtain a straight and solid L-shaped supporting structure (**Figure 10**).

The esthetic and functional results can be excellent, and damage at the donor site is normally minimal [19].

The auricular concha is instead insufficient, even when harvested bilaterally, for the correction of type III saddle nose, where marked dorsal depression and the absence of septal support are often combined with the lack of support from the nasal bones. All this is almost invariably accompanied by contraction of the skin and mucus membrane of a cicatricial nature or as a result of cocaine abuse or previous rhinoplasty.

The therapeutic approach to type III saddle nose is therefore aimed at the reconstruction of a sturdy L-shaped supporting structure capable of adequately withstanding the wound healing traction of the skin and mucus. The material of choice for the graft is unquestionably costal cartilage, shaped primarily with a view to reconstructing the caudal and dorsal support of the septum. To this end, it is possible

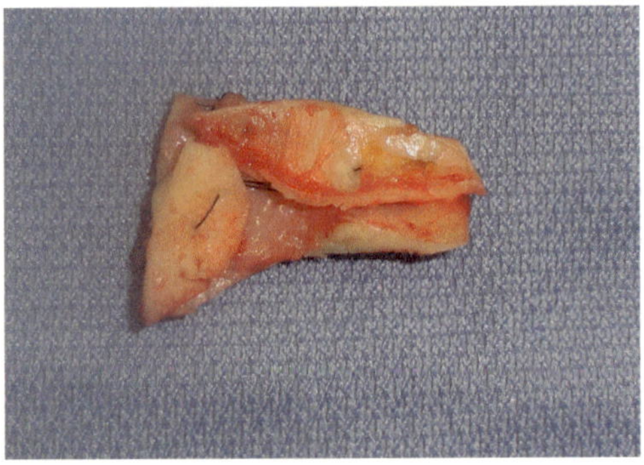

Figure 10.
Neoseptum totally reconstructed by conchal cartilage.

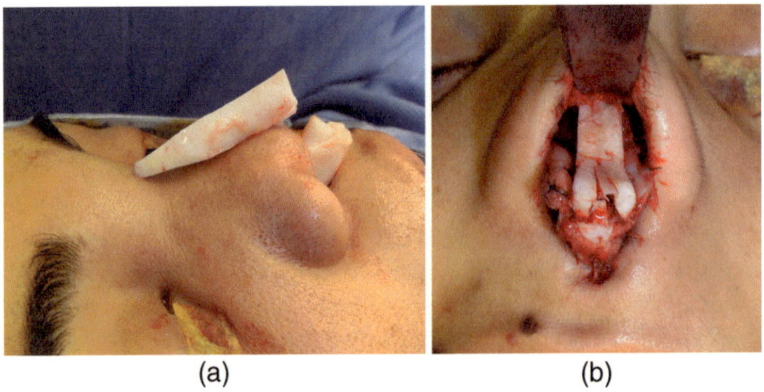

Figure 11.
(a) and (b) Antero-caudal septal structure reconstructed by costal cartilage.

to connect two pieces of a single rib (or two ribs), one to serve as the dorsal pillar with a socket to secure the other serving as the caudal pillar (**Figure 11a** and **b**).

It is not easy to secure the graft in place, above all in the cephalic portion. While some authors suggest that the creation of a pouch large enough for insertion of the graft is sufficient, others maintain that greater stability is required. According to Gunter et al., Kirschner thread can be used both to prevent distortion of the costal cartilage and to secure the graft cephalically [9]. Meyer suggests securing the graft with wire to the glabellar region after drilling a hole in the bone by means of open access [20]. Other authors maintain that it is sufficient to suture the graft to the skin above transcutaneously for 7–10 days. In the caudal portion, the graft should be secured with non-resorbable thread to the inferior nasal spine or its periosteum.

2. Summary

The saddle nose deformity is a big challenge for the surgeon. Its correction should be structural because the camouflage does not permit to correct the functional problems related to this pathology. In this chapter, we reviewed the different aspects of the saddle nose including its etiology, classification, and surgical treatment. The classification is very important because it can guide the surgical approach we should use for the correction. A fundamental diagnostic finding is the presence of the nasal septum which represents the gold material for the reconstruction. If this is missing, our reconstruction choice should be focused on auricular cartilage or costal cartilage in more severe cases.

Personal considerations of the author

The saddle nose represents one of the most challenging nasal deformities for the surgeon. The patient affected by saddle nose has almost always psychological problems, including concerns related to their own identity. The surgeon should evaluate the patient from different points of view, including diagnostic, therapeutical, and psychological. The choice of the correct surgical approach should be rational and based on the severity of the deformity. Different techniques of surgical correction of the saddle nose have to be present in our armamentarium, because only if we choose the right one, we can obtain optimal results.

Author details

Marianetti Tito Matteo
Marianetti Med Clinic, Rome, Italy

*Address all correspondence to: titomatteo.marianetti@tin.it

References

[1] Converse J. Reconstructive Plastic Surgery. 2nd ed. Vol. 2. Philadelphia PA: WB Saunders; 1977. p. 1141

[2] Tardy EM, Schwartz M, Parras G. Saddle nose deformity: Autogenous graft repair. Facial Plastic Surgery. 1989;**6**:2-21

[3] Mowlen R. Bone grafting. British Journal of Plastic Surgery. 1963;**16**:293-299

[4] Rozner L. Augmentation rhinoplasty. British Journal of Plastic Surgery. 1980;**33**:377-382

[5] Gunter JP, Rohrich RJ, Hackney FL. Dorsal augmentation: Onlay grafting using shake autologous septal cartilage. In: Dallas Rhinoplasty. Nasal Surgery by the Masters. 2nd ed. St Louis, MO: Quality Medical Publishing; 2007

[6] Fry H. Cartilage and cartilage grafts: The basic properties of the tissue and the components responsible for them. Plastic and Reconstructive Surgery. 1967;**40**:426-435

[7] Gibson T, Davis WB. The distortion of autogenous cartilage grafts: Its cause and prevention. British Journal of Plastic Surgery. 1958;**10**:257-268

[8] De Jong JH. Rib Graft in the Treatment of Saddle Deformity. Presented at the European Academy of Facial Surgery, London; 1983

[9] Gunter JP, Clark CP III, Friedmann RM, Hackney FL. Internal stabilization of large autologous rib cartilage grafts to avoid warping in rhinoplasty. In: Dallas Rhinoplasty. Nasal Surgery by the Masters. 2nd ed. St Louis, MO: Quality Medical Publishing; 2007

[10] Marin VP, Landecker A, Gunter JP. Harvesting rib cartilage grafts for secondary rhinoplasty. In: Dallas Rhinoplasty. Nasal Surgery by the Masters. 2nd ed. St Louis, MO: Quality Medical Publishing; 2007

[11] Gibson T. Cartilage grafts. British Medical Bulletin. 1965;**21**:153-165

[12] Milward TM. The fate of silastic and vitrathene nasal implants. British Journal of Plastic Surgery. 1972;**25**:1276-1278

[13] Deva AK, Merten S, Chang L. Silicone in nasal augmentation rhinoplasty: A decade of clinical experience. Plastic and Reconstructive Surgery. 1998 Sep;**102**(4):1230-1237

[14] Marvin JA. The application of cantilever bridge principle to silastic nasal support. British Journal of Plastic Surgery. 1980;**33**:404-406

[15] Mackay IS, Bull TR. The fate of silastic in the management of saddle deformity of the nose. The Journal of Laryngology and Otology. 1983;**97**:43-47

[16] Trenité N, Rhinoplasty GJ. A Practical Guide to Functional and Aesthetic Surgery of the Nose. The Netherlands: Kugler Publications; 2005

[17] Romo T, Slafani AB, Sabini P. Reconstruction of the major saddle nose deformity using composite allo-implants. Facial Plastic Surgery. 1998;**14**(2):151-157

[18] Daniel RK, Brenner KA. Saddle nose deformity: A new classification and treatment. Facial Plastic Surgery Clinics of North America. 2006;**14**(8):301-312

[19] Boccieri A. Subtotal reconstruction of the nasal septum using a conchal reshaped graft. Annals of Plastic Surgery. 2004;**53**(2):118-125

[20] Meyer R, Kesselring UK. Reconstructive surgery of the nose. Clinics in Plastic Surgery. 1981;**8**:435-446

Section 4

Rhinoplasty in Comorbidity

Chapter 5

Cleft Lip and Palate Patient Rhinoplasty

Angelo Cuzalina and Ahmed Tamim

Abstract

Cleft lip and palate patients represent one of the most difficult groups of patients for septorhinoplasty. Prior surgery at younger ages resulting in severe scar tissue is a major obstacle in most cleft rhinoplasties along with substantial asymmetries especially in the unilateral cleft patient. Replacement of missing and asymmetric cartilages and even bone is a key component for rhinoplasty in the cleft patient. Use of very sturdy cartilage typically from rib is almost always required to adequately resist the fibrotic soft tissues in the noses. Plus, rib cartilage can be carved into ideal septal extension and batten grafts that are required.

Keywords: rhinoplasty, nose job, cleft palate, reconstruction, rib grafting, septal extension graft, batten graft

1. Introduction

Rhinoplasty is one of the complex surgical procedures as it deals with skin, cartilage and bone, and all of that is done in the middle of the face, which makes it very noticeable and less forgiving. Now, to do the procedure on a cleft lip and palate patient is twice as hard, since you must contend with asymmetry, deficient bone and soft tissue [1]. Primary and secondary cleft rhinoplasty may be necessary to achieve optimal esthetic results for patients. This chapter focuses mainly on the secondary or definitive rhinoplasty reconstructive surgery to repair CLP and new techniques stressing the importance of robust septal extension grafts and batten grafts along with a novel method of placement.

2. Anatomy

2.1 Nasal deformity associated with unilateral cleft defect

The interrupted insertion of orbicularis oris muscle into the columella on the noncleft side forces the premaxilla, columella and caudal nasal septum towards that side [2, 3]. At the same time, as the orbicularis oris inserts into the alar base on the cleft side, the base is pulled laterally, inferiorly and posteriorly [2, 3]. The malformed lower lateral cartilage on the side of the cleft contributes majorly to the deformity of the nasal tip, causing it to be more blunt [2] (**Figure 1**). A shorter medial crus and a longer lateral crus on the cleft side results in a horizontally wider and displaced nostril on the cleft side [2, 3] (**Figure 2**).

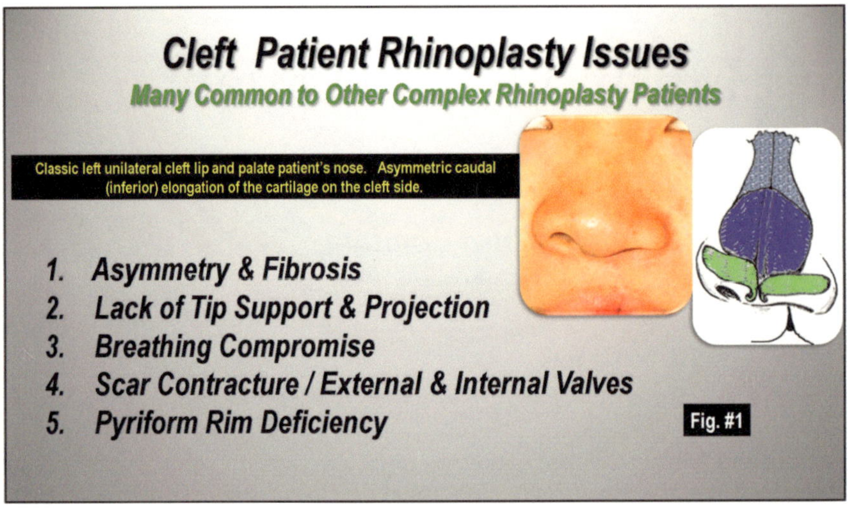

Figure 1.
Typical cleft lip and palate nasal issues are listed. Typically, a malformed lower lateral cartilage exists on the side of the cleft that contributes to the deformity of the nasal tip, causing it to be more flat and blunt.

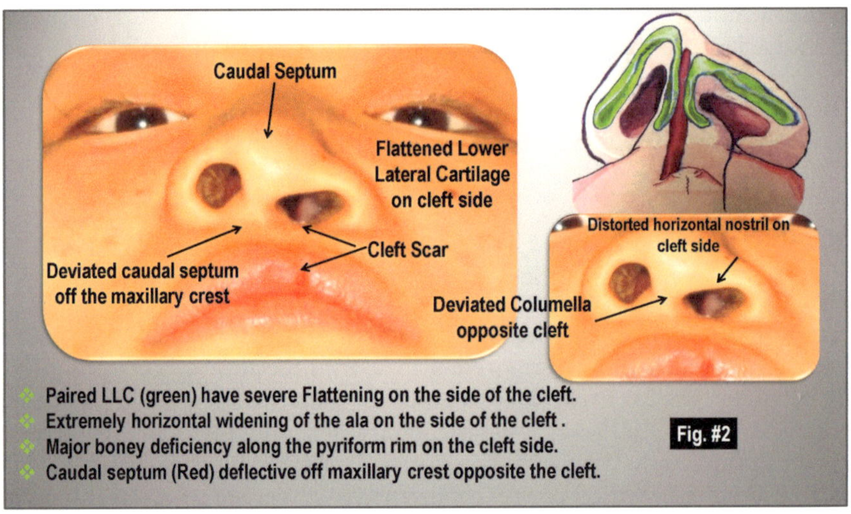

Figure 2.
A shorter medial crus and a longer lateral crus exist on the cleft side resulting in a horizontally wider and displaced nostril on the cleft side. The deficient pyriform rim bone can also be seen on the cleft side.

It is also worth noting that while the caudal septum is forced towards the noncleft side, the rest of the septum is deviated towards the cleft side. This septal bowing, along with decreased nasal aperture, causes nasal air obstruction.

Moreover, internal vestibular webbing is evident on the cleft side causing the nostril margin on that side to buckle inwardly [3].

Also, the lower lateral cartilage in introverted which cause further nasal obstruction by narrowing the external nasal valve and makes the nasal ala look thicker and hooded [2]. The introversion of the lower lateral cartilage, secondary to the pressure from the abnormal position of the alar base, and columella which push the cartilage down and back [4] (**Figure 3**). The asymmetries of the LLC and Septum requires a specific treatment most commonly involving asymmetric lateral crural steal techniques fixated to a septal extension graft (**Figures 4** and **5**).

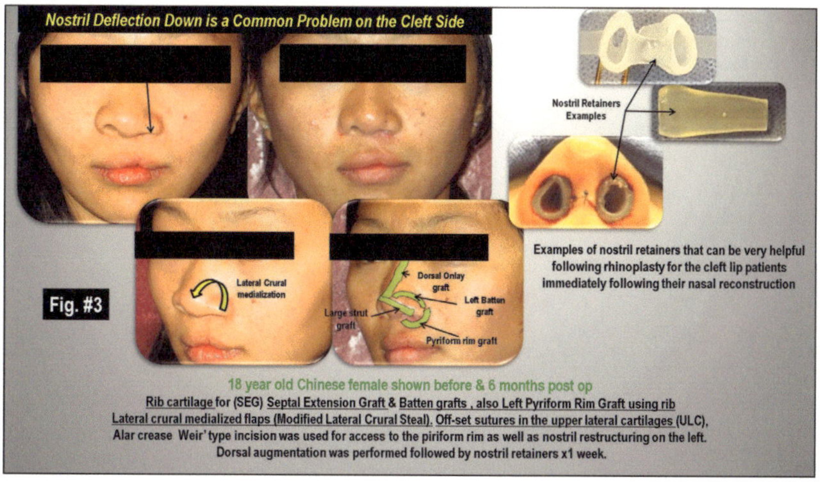

Figure 3.
Before and 6 months after classic rhinoplasty surgery to improve the patient's nose who has a left cleft lip and palate. Multiple grafts are required, particularly septal extension, batten, and pyriform rim grafts.

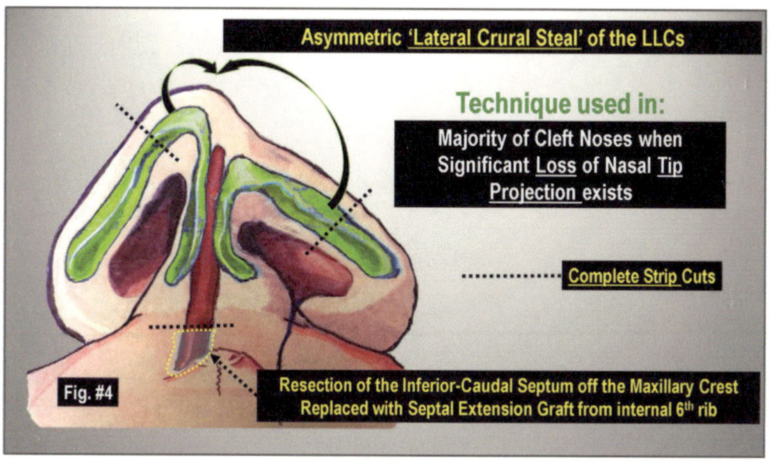

Figure 4.
The asymmetric of the LLC and septum requires a specific treatment shown involving an asymmetric lateral crural steal rotation cartilage flaps fixated to a septal extension graft.

2.2 Nasal deformity associated with bilateral cleft defect

Bilateral and unilateral nasal cleft deformities are similar and share many characteristics [3]. However, bilateral nasal cleft defects tend to be symmetrical [2]. The shortness, or in some cases, the absence of the columella is caused by soft tissue deficiency between the nasal tip and upper lip [2] (**Figure 6**).

Absence of nasal floor with bilateral hypoplastic maxilla is another key feature of bilateral nasal cleft deformity [3]. The alar base is wide and positioned caudally, laterally and inferiorly, with less defined nasal tip due to the longer lateral crus and shorted medial crus of the lower lateral cartilage on cleft side [2, 3]. Vestibular webbing is seen bilaterally [3].

The septum is typically straight in the midline due to the symmetry. However, in some cases where there is asymmetry, the less affected side applies more force to the caudal septum pulling it towards that side [2, 3].

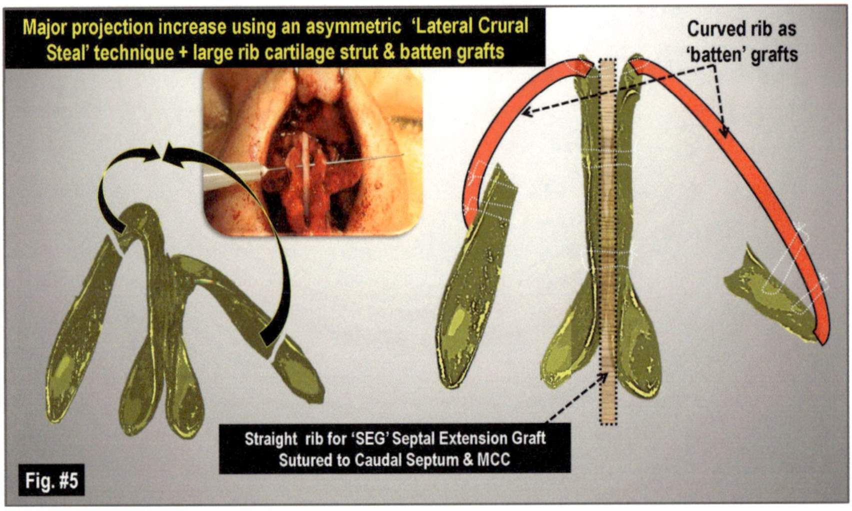

Figure 5.
Diagrams show the attachment of the asymmetric rotation of the lower lateral cartilage flaps to both large septal extension graft and as curved batten graft for recreation of normal lower nose architecture.

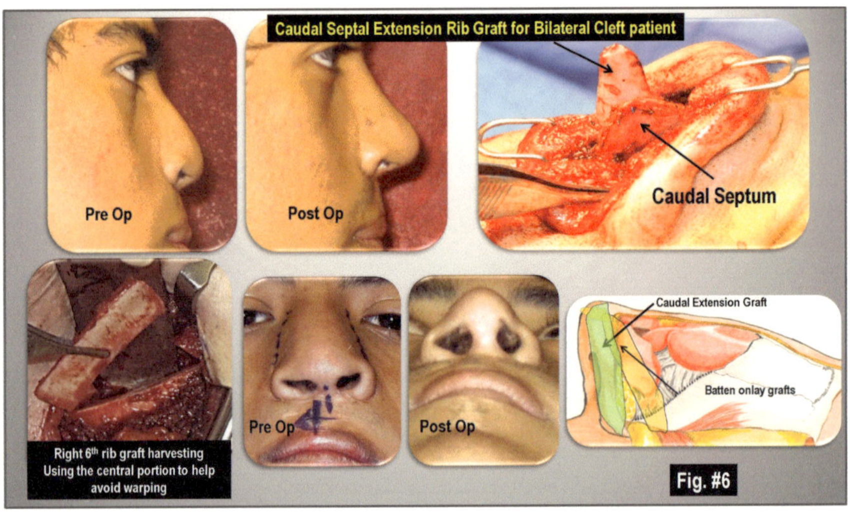

Figure 6.
A short columella is caused by soft tissue deficiency between the nasal tip and upper lip, especially in some bilateral cleft cases as shown. Large and strong septal extension grafts from rib are particularly important for these cases.

2.3 Surgical timing

Surgical nasal deformity repair is normally done in multiple stages, divided based on surgical timing: primary, intermediate, and secondary. Primary rhinoplasty is performed at the time of cleft lip repair [4–6]. The typical age of cleft lip repair is 2–3 months old [4, 7]. However, current mainstream surgical timing remains around 3 months of age to avoid higher risk of complications, especially during anesthesia [7].

Intermediate rhinoplasty is performed at age 5–11 years old, typically between 4 and 6 years old before patients attend school [2, 5]. And lastly, secondary or definitive rhinoplasty is generally undergone after completion of facial growth, which differs based on gender [2]. For females it is usually 14–16 years of age, while males it is later at 16–18 years of age [2]. However, there are other factors that can contribute to the timing of the definitive rhinoplasty, including: patient's size, extent of deformity, and situations may warrant definitive rhinoplasty as early as age 10-12 in limited situations [6].

2.4 Primary rhinoplasty

Rhinoplasty performed at this stage is currently considered by many surgeons as the accepted surgical treatment [4]. It is even considered the standard of care in the United States amongst other countries [8]. The original notion that primary rhinoplasty can interfere with facial growth has been disputed by many recent studies [2].

The primary target of this surgery is to obtain a symmetrical nasal tip and alar base [4]. There are many described techniques to correct the asymmetrical unilateral nasal deformity, including V-Y-Z plasty [2, 9]. In general, the lower lateral cartilage is released and repositioned [2–4, 6]. The alar base is separated from the pyriform aperture and maxilla to be repositioned symmetrically [4, 6]. Nasal tip plasty is performed to enhance its projection [4]. Moreover, caudal nasal septum is repaired at this stage by attaching it to the anterior nasal spine [2]. The usage of presurgical nasoalveolar molding (NAM) device can be successful in shaping nasal cartilage within the first 6 weeks after birth, when the cartilage is more elastic due to high levels of circulating maternal estrogen [10].

2.5 Intermediate rhinoplasty

This surgery is only performed when needed. Some bilateral cleft nasal deformity patients undergo surgery at this stage to correct severely asymmetrical nasal tip that was not repaired in primary rhinoplasty [2, 6]. It also aims at lengthening shortened columella [6]. For unilateral nasal deformities, its addresses any residual defects in lower lateral cartilage and lateral vestibular webbing.

Septal repositioning and cartilage grafting are not done at this stage; they are postponed until complete skeletal growth is achieved in adulthood [2].

2.6 Secondary/definitive

It is usually needed to correct secondary deformities and scarring developing after primary cleft lip and nose repair. The success of primary rhinoplasty and the severity of secondary deformities are dependent on surgeon's skill and experience [8].

Open approach is the most common technique used in definitive rhinoplasty, as it allows for enhanced exposure of muscle structure, cartilage, vestibular lining, and dense scarring [2, 4, 6]. It also aids in precise positioning of lateral lower cartilage, nasal base, and septum, as well as accurate grafting and suturing [6].

Goals of definitive rhinoplasty include: nasal and tip definition, removal of scar and fibrofatty tissue, and nasal obstruction repair [4, 6] (**Figure 7**). In some cases, depending on the complexity of the cleft lip and palate deformity, Le Forte maybe needed to correct secondary maxillary hypoplasia [11]. Definitive rhinoplasty is typically performed after repairing major skeletal defects with necessary orthognathic surgery [3].

2.7 Incision

Secondary cleft rhinoplasty is almost always performed via an open approach, giving access to different parts of the nose that needs reconstruction along with direct visualization. The usual incision is infracartilaginous and V or W shaped transcolumellar. Keep in mind that the medial crura are right under the skin in the lateral portion of the columella, so a superficial dissection is indicated at this area [2]. Once the skin flap is elevated, the cartilage and bone components can be examined thoroughly.

2.8 Septum

Deviated septum in cleft patients causes airway obstruction by causing physical stenosis and turbulent airflow [12]. Correcting the septum involves dissecting its cartilaginous and bony parts, including the vomer and perpendicular plate of the ethmoid bone (PPE) [12]. However, it is best to maintain at least 1-cm width of dorsal and caudal septal segments, or L-strut, to preserve the tip and dorsal nasal support [2]. There should also be more than 40% fixation area, or contact point, between nasal crest of maxilla and L-strut when dissecting caudal septum [2]. This decreases the strain energy and stress values on septum, and relieves excessive load forces on L-strut, which lessens the chances of future nasal deformities, including collapse of dorsal septum or saddle deformity, and nasal tip ptosis [2]. However, in some cases, the septal deviation is severe enough that the dissection of the deviated segment and its replacement with a straight graft becomes necessary. The graft is obtained from septal cartilage, or the rib cartilage maybe used if a larger segment is needed [13]. Sutures through the upper lateral cartilages and septum are placed to apply force in the opposite direction of the L-strut deviation, and thus correcting it and creating symmetry [14].

In certain cases, a notch is made in the nasal spine using a straight osteotome to allow for a stronger attachment of the caudal strut [15].

Spreader grafts and batten onlay grafts can be harvested from the resected parts of the quadrangular septal cartilage, but most often from the curved portion of the right sixth rib in order to have adequate shape, size and strength of cartilage required in the cleft rhinoplasty [3] (**Figure 8**). For instance, curved batten grafts are sutured to the lower lateral cartilage and strut to take the natural convex form of the external nasal valve and support it [3].

The transcolumellar open incision is the most common access technique in definitive rhinoplasty as it provides better exposure of the septal cartilage [16]. The incision is made anterior to the footplate segments of the medial crura of the lower lateral cartilage [16]. A mucoperichondrial flap is raised with caution not to perforate the surrounding mucosa to allow excellent coverage of a large SEG from rib [3].

2.9 Spreader graft

Spreader grafts are used to open up the internal nasal valve, mainly the middle third of the nose and improve the breathing [3, 12]. They are usually obtained from either the nasal septal cartilage or part of the harvested rib cartilage. They are placed between the septum and upper lateral cartilage bilaterally and secured with sutures [12]. If needed, the spreader graft can extend more caudally and act as a strut graft for better nasal tip support and it also helps with the septum stability and straightening. Spreader grafts can sometimes be used to correct severe septal deviation, by placing the grafts along the dorsal septum, while reattaching the caudal strut to the nasal spine between the medial crura by suture fixation[17–21].

2.10 Nasal and dorsum osteotomies

The nasal dorsum in cleft patient is usually deficient and flat and an easy was to address that is applying a silicone implant or using a dorsal onlay graft from rib (**Figure 9**). Septum and nasal bones usually deviate towards the non-cleft side, as the root of the nasal dorsum is deviated towards the cleft site [2]. If a dorsal hump existed, reduction of the bone by rasping and cartilage by either no. 15 blade or a scissor will be needed. Usually after the reduction, patient will develop an open roof deformity and to treat that, a lateral nasal osteotomy is required to narrow the width. A small 2–3 mm osteotome is utilized to create micro punctures along the planned cut and the osteotome is inserted percutaneous or preferably transnasally and usually the osteotomies are done low to high [2] (**Figure 10**).

2.11 Nasal tip, lower lateral cartilage and sturdy batten grafts

The lower lateral cartilage on the cleft side is usually collapsed vertically and displaced inferiorly. And to address and correct the lower lateral cartilages, an open

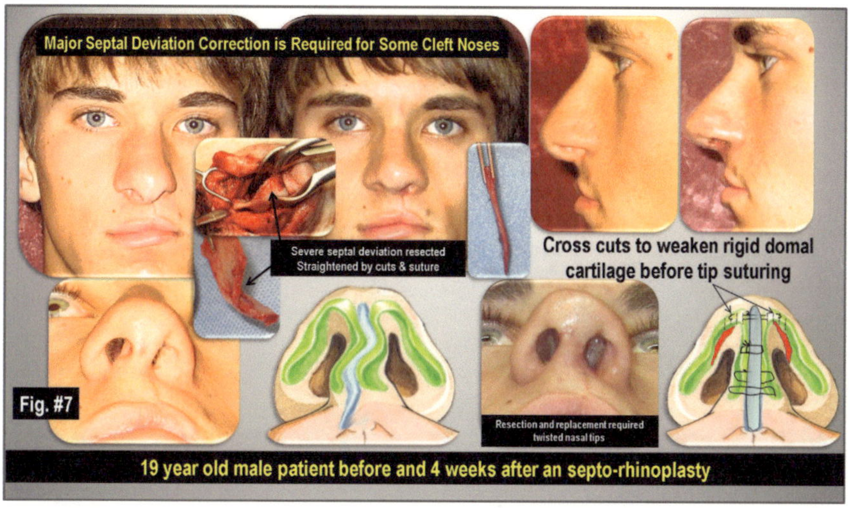

Figure 7.
This figure demonstrates the importance of septal extension grafts to correct major tip and caudal septal deviation in cleft patients. The severely deviated cartilage often must be completely removed and replaced with new grafted cartilage.

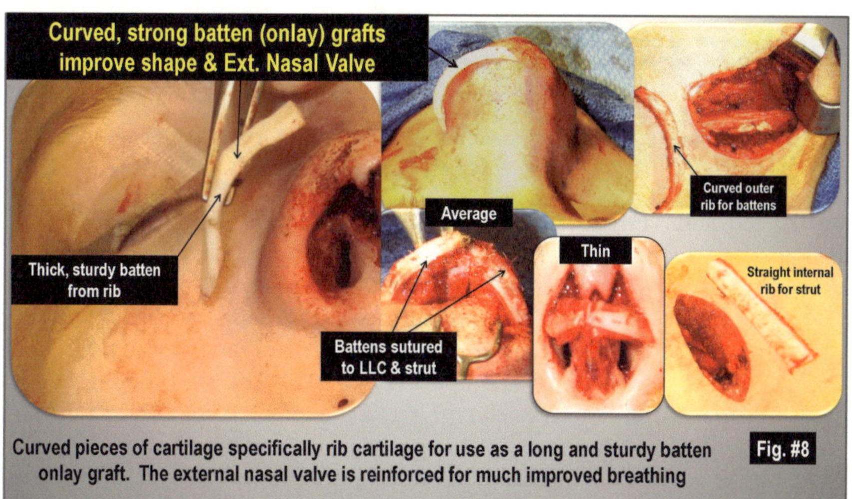

Figure 8.
Curved batten onlay grafts are demonstrated. Spreader grafts and batten onlay grafts can be harvested from the resected parts of the quadrangular septal cartilage, but most often from the curved portion of the right sixth rib.

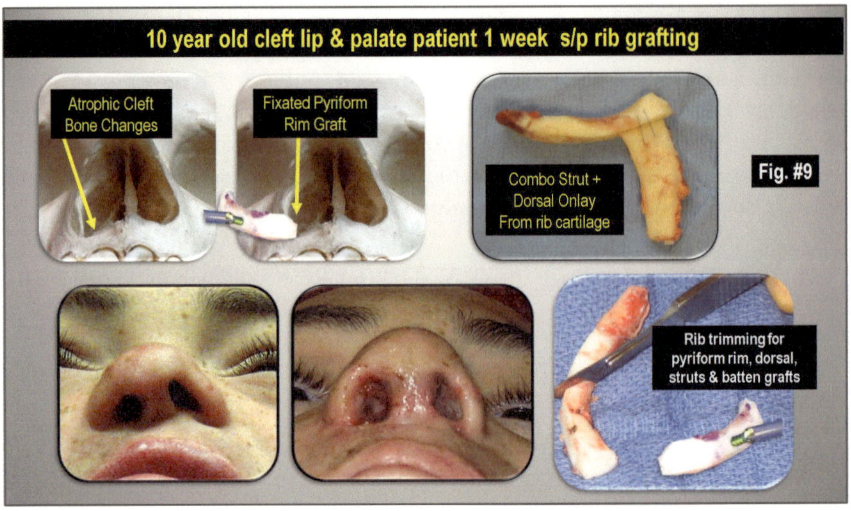

Figure 9.
A deficient and flat nasal dorsum in a cleft patient can be addressed by using a dorsal onlay graft from rib as demonstrated. The same rib can also be used for augmentation of the deficient pyriform rim.

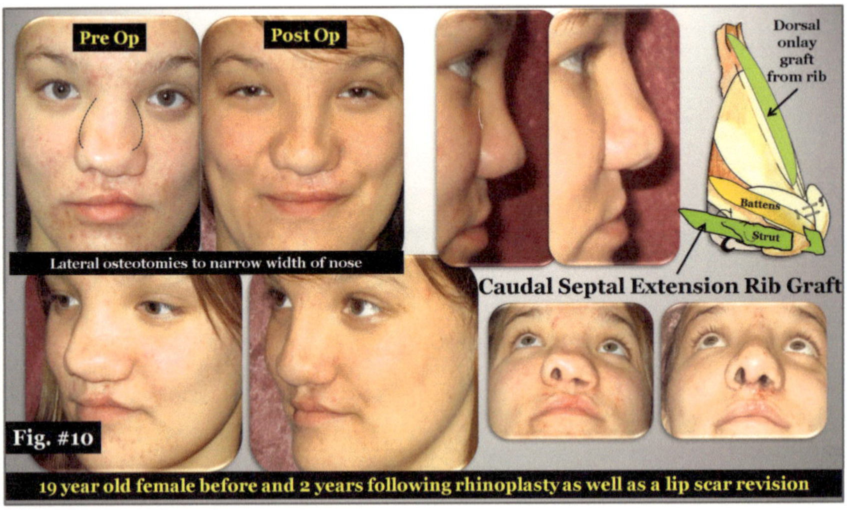

Figure 10.
A small 2–3 mm osteotome is utilized to create micropunctures along the planned osteotomies as shown. The cleft patient may still require dorsal grafting along with the osteotomies in some cases.

rhinoplasty incision is utilized, cephalic trimming of the cartilage is performed if LLC are too large, making sure to leave at least 5 mm for support. Next, the septum can be accessed through transdomal dissection and then repair the septum and harvest cartilage, if no rib cartilage harvest is planned/needed; a caudal septum extension graft is placed and secured to the lower lateral cartilage and the septum, which will improve the nasal tip projection and support (**Figure 11**). The graft should be slightly behind the medial crura, otherwise the columella can look too wide or simply feel too firm to the patient [13]. Extra strengthening of the nasal base can be done by applying mattress sutures holding the medial crural cartilage to the septum and positioning the tip in a more cephalic location [13]. To achieve better symmetry to the nasal tip, a lateral crural steal or advancement flap is used [3] (**Figures 4** and **5**). Where a longer part of the lateral crus on the cleft side is cut and a shorter part of the lateral crus on the non-cleft side is cut as the cleft side lateral crus cartilage is longer horizontally and shorter vertically at the medial crus than the non-cleft side and that will allow for more symmetry and tip projection. Then a rib cartilage graft is used to reconstruct bilateral lower lateral cartilage crus which can be placed as a batten only or below the remaining lateral crus. Long, strong batten grafts are often a critical component to success especially if alar retraction exist (**Figure 12**). If further tip projection is needed, a shield graft can be utilized. For a good tip support, the caudal septum extension graft needs to extend past the septum for a minimum of 4–5 mm with a thickness of at least 1 mm. The cartilage harvested from the septum can be used for that or if more needed a rib cartilage can be used, which is more common in for the cleft rhinoplasty cases as the thickness of the cartilage provide enough resistance to hold the post inflammatory changes, besides most of the time there will be multiple areas of deficiencies to be addressed and the septal cartilage would not be enough to cover all of them.

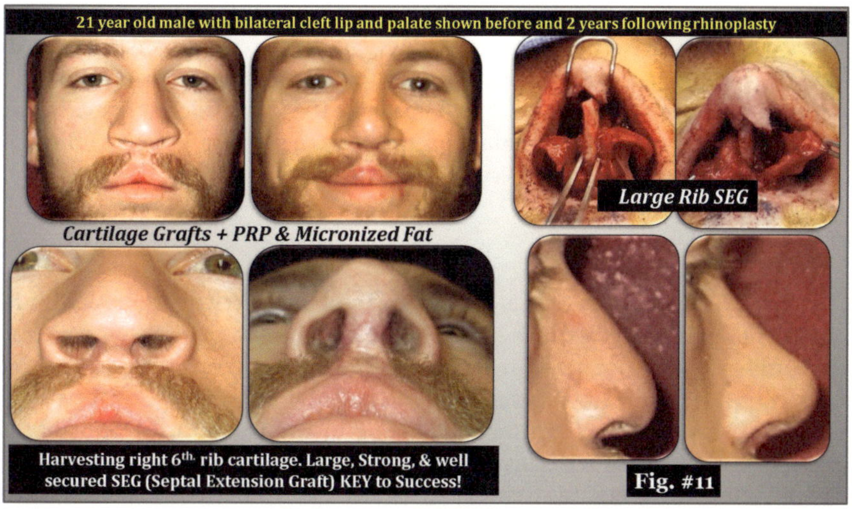

Figure 11.
The septum is accessed and shown via a transdomal dissection followed by placement of a caudal septum extension secured to the lower lateral cartilage and the septum. This dramatically improves the nasal tip projection and support.

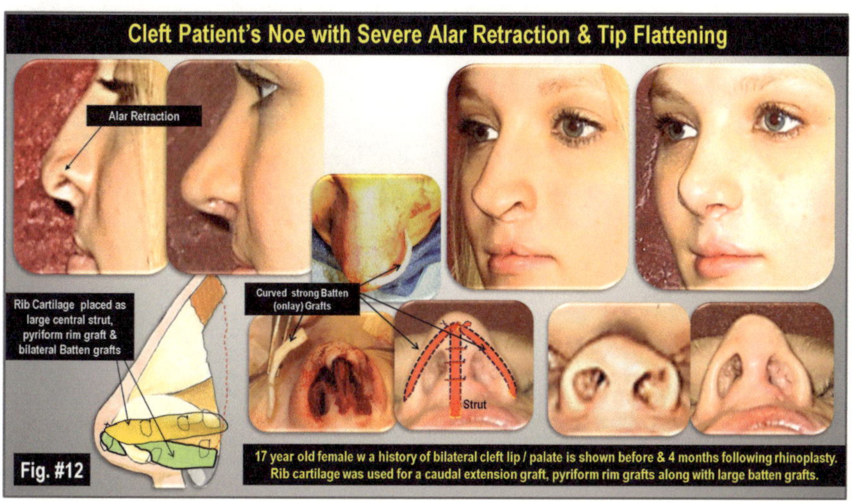

Figure 12.
Long, strong batten grafts often are a critical component to success and demonstrated in this figure. They are especially useful if alar retraction exists prior to the rhinoplasty.

2.12 Piriform rim and premaxilla augmentation

Cleft lip and palate patients will have piriform rim deficiency, which leads to inferior and posterior displacement of the nose at the side of the cleft, and if left unaddressed will lead to asymmetric results, even if all the other aspects of the rhinoplasty were well addressed [3]. Part of the rib graft can be used and stacked for augmentation and secured with a screw, other options are silicone implant, cortical bone or fat grafting [2] (**Figure 9**).

2.13 Alar base reduction

The last portion of the rhinoplasty is to address the alar base. Usually it is inferiorly and laterally displaced (**Figure 13**). To fix the asymmetry V-Y advancement or the weir procedure (alar resection) are utilized at the alar facial groove [3]. The weir procedure is generally used when there is lateral skin excess and also that will provide an access to the piriform rim for augmentation (**Figure 14**). It is recommended to use nostril retainer to help shape the nasal sill. Skin grafting or composite grafting just inside the ala is performed when enlargement of the nostril size is required to improve symmetry (**Figure 15**).

2.14 Rib cartilage

Compared to autologous tissue, alloplastic implants carry higher risk of infection and dehiscence. Rib cartilage is the source of choice in patients who need larger sturdy grafts to repair severe deformities of nasal tip projection and provide strong support. Its main advantages include its availability in large quantities if needed, resistance of scar contracture, strength, and versatility. Donor site morbidity is one of its main disadvantages, including post-surgical pain, scarring, and risk of pneumothorax. In some cases, especially in older populations, rib cartilage graft can ossify. In other cases, graft warping has been documented [3]. The graft is typically harvested from the sixth or seventh rib, usually the right side.

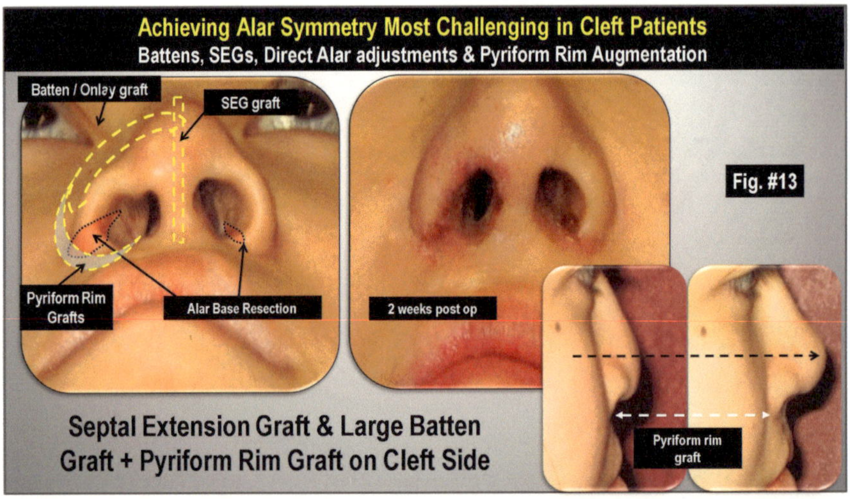

Figure 13.
The last portion of the rhinoplasty addressed is the alar base shown. The base on the cleft side is often inferiorly and laterally displaced. The weir procedure is generally used when there is lateral skin excess and provides an access to the piriform rim for augmentation.

Incision is made with a 10 blade, and electrocautery is used for dissection through subcutaneous tissue and muscle to access the rib, and then incise through the perichondrium.

The subperichondral dissection extends from the junction of the sternum and cartilage to the osseocartilaginous junction, and is carried posteriorly. To protect the perichondrium, it is best to place a retractor posterior to the rib. It is worth noting that full rib resection or discontinuous harvesting should be avoided to decrease post-op complications. The middle portion of rim is used for the SEG to avoid warpage and soaked in sterile saline for 1 h prior to placement. In some severe deformities where a large graft is needed, harvesting cartilage from more than one rib maybe indicated. After wound irrigation and obtaining hemostasis, it is imperative to rule out pneumothorax by filling donor site with saline and having anesthesia provider

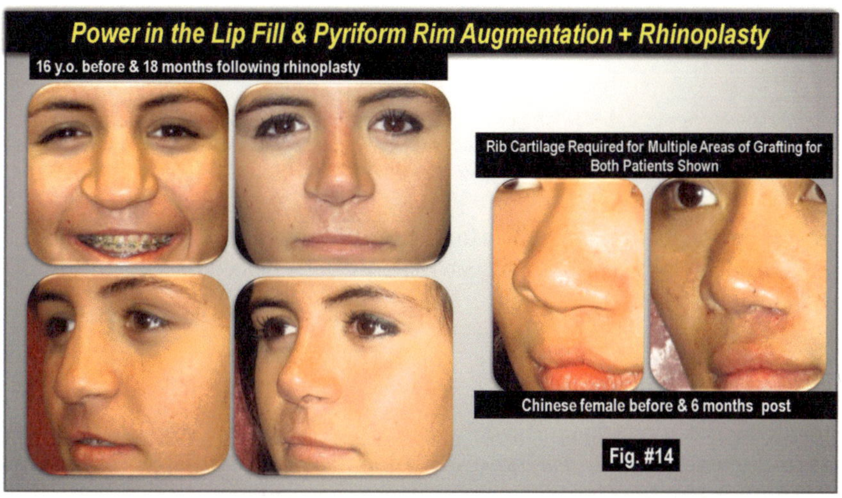

Figure 14.
Augmentation of the deficient pyriform rim as well the deficient lip and scar provides an excellent final refinement for the rhinoplasty procedure in the cleft lip patient.

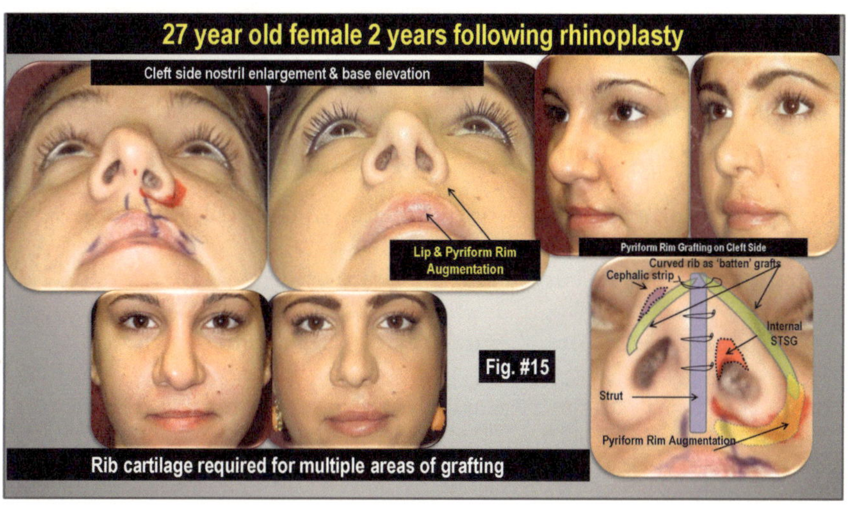

Figure 15.
Skin grafting or composite grafting just inside the ala is occasionally required when enlargement of the nostril size is required to improve symmetry or to prevent nostril stenosis in restricted or previously operated cases.

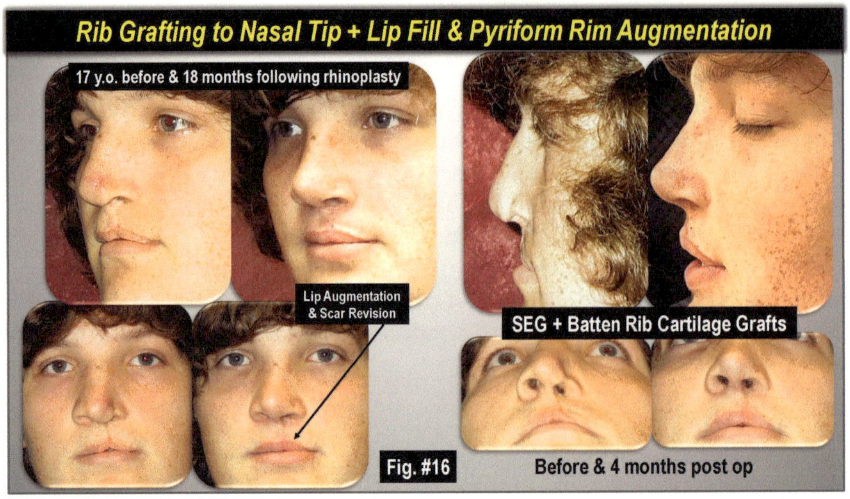

Figure 16.
Enhancing the appearance of a deficient lip or philtral ridge on the cleft side can greatly improve the overall results during rhinoplasty for the cleft lip and palate patient. The patient shown had augmentation to all the above areas in addition to the typical nasal cartilage grafting.

apply positive pressure to lungs. Any indication of lung perforation will need to be addressed immediately. Then, a collagen matrix can be placed to obliterate the dead space, along with layered suturing.

2.15 Lip and philtral ridge

Enhancing the appearance of a deficient lip or philtral ridge on the cleft side can greatly improve the overall results during rhinoplasty for the cleft lip and palate patient (**Figure 16**). Various fillers exist that can be used under a flat philtral ridge or atrophic portion of the lip. Also, fat grafting via newer micronized fat injection systems like ALMI® give the surgeon the ability to be much more precise with fat injections. The growth factors and pre adipocytes also may improve internal scar softness beyond that which can be done by a formal scar revision.

3. Conclusion

Key new points for technique:

- Septal extension grafts made from the interior of rib cartilage (**Figures 6** and **11**).
- Batten grafts from the curved portion of rib cartilage (**Figures 8** and **12**).
- Modified asymmetric lateral crural steal plus rib (**Figures 4** and 5).
- Large fixated pyriform rim/premaxilla bone or cartilage grafting (**Figures 9** and **15**).

Even though cleft rhinoplasty is a complex surgical procedure, its results can be satisfying for the surgeon and life changing for the patients as it provides symmetry, improved esthetics and enhanced functionality, including better breathing. Its complexity originates from the need of multiple surgical stages over the years, which require a full surgical team from different specialties. Major cartilaginous grafting is typicallyneeded for definitive rhinoplasty to repair nasal tip projection and septal deviation. Rib cartilage grafts are better compared to other donor sites, due to its strength, large supply when needed, ease of shaping, and high resistance to scar contracture. Moreover, rib cartilage grafts for nasal tip repair, may also be used rather than piriform rim implants in cases of premaxilla and piriform rim deficiency which must be addressed for best results.

Author details

Angelo Cuzalina[1*] and Ahmed Tamim[2]

1 AACS Cosmetic Surgery Fellowship Program, Tulsa Surgical Arts, Tulsa, OK, USA

2 Tulsa Surgical Arts, Tulsa, OK, USA

*Address all correspondence to: angelo@tulsasurgicalarts.com

References

[1] Bendre DV, Ofodile FA. Rhinoplasty in adolescent cleft patients. Oral and Maxillofacial Surgery Clinics of North America. 2002;**14**(4):453-461

[2] Kaufman Y et al. Cleft nasal deformity and rhinoplasty. Seminars in Plastic Surgery. 2012;**26**(4):184-190

[3] Cuzalina A, Jung C. Rhinoplasty for the cleft lip and palate patient. Oral and Maxillofacial Surgery Clinics of North America. 2016;**28**(2):189-202

[4] Gabriel M-C, Carlos M-M. Chapter 1: Cleft lip nasal deformity: Analysis and treatment. In: Advances of Plastic and Reconstructive Surgery. Open Access Books. Available at: http://openaccessebooks.com/plastic-reconstructive-surgery/cleft-lip-nasal-deformity-analysis-and-treatment.pdf [Accessed: August 25, 2018]

[5] Baskaran M et al. Cleft rhinoplasty. Journal of Pharmacy & Bioallied Sciences. 2015;**2**(Suppl 2):S691-S694

[6] Sykes JM, Senders CW. Surgery of the cleft lip and nasal deformity. Operative Techniques in Otolaryngology-Head and Neck Surgery. 1990;**1**(4):219-224

[7] Berkowitz S. Lip and palate surgery. In: Berkowitz S, editor. Cleft lip and Palate: Diagnosis and Management. New York: Springer; 2006. pp. 315-351

[8] Slayer KE et al. Unilateral cleft lip—Approach and technique. Seminars in Plastic Surgery. 2005;**19**(4):313-328

[9] Rossell-Perry P. Primary unilateral cleft lip nasal deformity repair using V-Y-Z plasty: An anthropometric study. Indian Journal of Plastic Surgery. 2017;**50**(2):180-186

[10] Subramanian CS et al. A modified presurgical orthopedic (nasoalveolar molding) device in the treatment of unilateral cleft lip and palate. European Journal of Dentistry. 2016;**10**(3):435-438

[11] Good PM, Mulliken JB, Padwa BL. Frequency of Le Fort I osteotomy after repaired cleft lip and palate or cleft palate. The Cleft Palate-Craniofacial Journal. 2007;**44**(4):396-401

[12] Ingels KJAO, Orhan KS, van Heerbeek N. The effect of spreader grafts on nasal dorsal width in patients with nasal valve insufficiency. Archives of Facial Plastic Surgery. 2008;**10**(5):354-356

[13] Guyuron B. MOC-PS(SM) CME article: Late cleft lip nasal deformity. Plastic and Reconstructive Surgery. 2008;**121**(4, Suppl):1-11

[14] Teymoortash A, Fasunla JA, Sazgar AA. The value of spreader grafts in rhinoplasty: A critical review. European Archives of Oto-Rhino-Laryngology. 2012;**269**(5):1411-1416

[15] Saleh H, Khoury E. Closed rhinoplasty. In: Cheney ML, Hadlock TA, editors. Facial Surgery: Facial and Reconstructive. Florida: CRC Press; 2015. pp. 337-364

[16] Petropoulos I, Karagiannidis K, Kontzoglou G. Our experience in open rhinoplasty. Hippokratia. 2007;**11**(1):35-38

[17] Jiri B et al. Successful early neonatal repair of cleft lip within first 8 days of life. International Journal of Pediatric Otorhinolaryngology. 2012;**76**(11):1616-1626

[18] Jahanbin A et al. Treatment approach for maxillary hypoplasia in cleft patients: Class III elastics with skeletal anchorage (Report of two cases). Iranian

Journal of Otorhinolaryngology. 2016;**28**(87):297-302

[19] Massie JP et al. Nasal septal anatomy in skeletally mature patients with cleft lip and palate. JAMA Facial Plastic Surgery. 2016;**18**(5):347-353

[20] Lee J-S et al. Redefining the septal L-strut in septal surgery. PLoS One. 2015. DOI: 10.1371/journal.pone.0119996

[21] Cerkes N. The crooked nose: Principles of treatment. Aesthetic Surgery Journal. 2011;**31**(2):241-257. DOI: 10.1177/1090820X10394167

Chapter 6

Surgery for Sleep-Disordered Breathing

Ken-ichi Hisamatsu, Hiroumi Matsuzaki, Itsuhiro Kudou and Kiyoshi Makiyama

Abstract

We evaluated the outcomes of nasal surgery for sleep-disordered breathing, including obstructive sleep apnea syndrome (OSAS), respiratory effort-related arousal, and snoring. To reduce pharyngeal negative pressure during sleep, the nasal parasympathetic nerve was resected, and the nasal cavity was enlarged by submucosal inferior turbinectomy and septoplasty if necessary. Of the 45 severe OSAS patients, symptoms were significantly ameliorated in 67%. This low-invasiveness nasal operation effectively reduced excessive daytime sleepiness and bothersome snoring without any pharyngeal operation. In addition, no side effects have been reported to be associated with this treatment regimen.

Keywords: nasal surgery, sleep-disordered breathing, snoring, hypersomnia, obstructive sleep apnea syndrome

1. Introduction

Sleep-disordered breathing (SDB) includes mild-to-severe obstructive apnea syndrome (OSAS), respiratory effort-related arousal (RERA), other hypersomnia, and socially unacceptable snoring. The pathophysiology of SDB involves nocturnal pharyngeal negative pressur, collapsibility of the soft palate, and an increased inspired air volume due to obesity, a narrow upper airway, and an oropharyngeal shape with a wide pillar and long uvula.

A number of patients suffer from excessive daytime sleepiness, bothersome snoring, and apnea pointed out by a member of their family or bed partner. Hypersomnia can cause traffic accidents and similar dangerous incidents, so this disorder should be managed quickly when it is noted. Furthermore, snoring affects the quality of life (QOL), especially in people who work in group settings, such as firefighters and police officers.

Septoplasty was reported to improve the QOL [1]. Nasal surgery can enlarge the nasal cavity, resulting in a reduction in the nasal resistance and subsequent amelioration of SDB. Generally, OSAS is managed with CPAP therapy. However, other SDBs are typically not managed this way either for financial reasons or due to the fact that they are not covered for CPAP by the Japanese National Insurance System.

At our institution, we use nasal surgery to reduce nocturnal nasal resistance.

The aim of this study was to clarify the efficacy of nasal surgery for resolving SDB.

2. Material and methods

Active anterior rhinomanometry was performed using a Spirometer HI-801 (Chest Co., Tokyo, Japan). PSG was performed using a PSG amplifier (Embla N7000; Natus Company, Pleasanton, CA, USA). OSAS was diagnosed according to the report of the American Academy of Sleep Medicine Task Force [2].

The nasal surgery comprised conventional septoplasty and bilateral submucosal inferior turbinectomy with posterior nasal neurectomy [3] and was performed under local anesthesia. Indications of this operation were unilateral and/or bilateral high nasal resistance (>0.35 Pa/cm^3/s), marked septal deviation, and marked protrusion of the inferior turbinate and hypertrophic mucosa. To protect the mucosal from damage, between a gauze coated with kichin (Beschitin®F; Nipro Co., Osaka, Japan), sandwiched bet pieces of gelatin sponge, was packed into the nasal cavity for 2 days.

The judging criteria were selected according to the findings of our previous report [4]. Daytime sleepiness was assessed by the Epworth sleepiness scale [5].

The study protocol was reviewed and approved by the ethics committees of Nihon University Hospital. This original retrospective study on the outcomes of nasal surgery for SDB was registered at the University Hospital Medical Information Network Clinical Trial Registry (identifier: UMIN 000011997; trial name: Effect of nasal surgery on sleep-disordered breathing).

3. Statistical analyses

The data were analyzed by using Wilcoxon matched-pair signed rank test, and a p value of <0.05 was considered to be significant.

4. Results

4.1 Subjects

The present study enrolled 52 patients with severe OSAS, 33 with moderate OSAS, 19 with mild OSAS, 45 with RERA, and 41 snorers. Patients' background details are shown in **Table 1**. All patients provided their informed consent before undergoing the nasal surgery.

	N	Sex	N	Age, mean(SD), year	BMI, (SD), kg/m^2
Severe OSAS	52	M	44	46.22 ± 10.85	26.37 ± 4.47
		F	8	47.5 ± 7.93	25.74 ± 2.79
Moderate OSAS	33	M	26	39.54 ± 11.29	24.31 ± 3.94
		F	7	46.43 ± 5.4	24.2 ± 5.09
Mild OSAS	19	M	13	44.23 ± 8.89	24.52 ± 2.74
		F	6	45.67 ± 8.21	24.88 ± 8.21
RERA	45	M	24	38.63 ± 10.99	23.35 ± 3.56
		F	21	36.81 ± 11.89	22.99 ± 4.46
Snorer	41	M	26	39.03 ± 12.76	24.53 ± 3.16
		F	15	47.4 ± 10.19	20.82 ± 2.61

Table 1.
Patient's background.

			OSAS		
			Highly effective	Effective	Ineffective
		Sex			
Severe OSAS	40	M	1	27(70%)	12
	5	F		4	1
Moderate OSAS	10	M		8	2
	5	F		4	1
Mild OSAS	3	M		2	1
	0	F		0	0

Table 2.
Effect of NS on sleep-disordered breathing.

4.2 Operative details

The outcomes of surgery are shown in **Tables 2** and **3**. Severe OSAS was ameliorated in 28 of the 40 male patients (70%) and 4 of the 5 female patients (80%) by nasal operation without any pharyngeal intervention. Moderate OSAS was ameliorated in 8 of the 10 male patients (80%) and 4 of the 5 female patients (80%) by nasal operation without any pharyngeal intervention (**Table 2**). The improvement rate of hypersomnia was particularly high in RERA patients (23 of 24 male patients [95.8%] and all 20 female patients [100%]), although the results of many studies remain unclear, and the snoring symptoms substantially improved 127/151 (84.1%) (**Table 3**). The improvement rate of all SDB was 111/140 (79.2%) for hypersomnia and 127/151 (84.1%) for snoring.

4.3 Findings of polysomnography

The preoperative and postoperative values of apnea index (AI), apnea hypopnea index (AHI), and $SpO_2 < 90\%$ were analyzed, with results shown in **Table 4**.

		Hypersomnia		Snore		Allergic rhinitis
		Effective	Obscure	Effective	Ineffective	Improved
	Sex					
Severe OSAS	M	30	19	31	6	6
	F	3	5	5	0	1
Moderate OSAS	M	13	1	18	4	2
	F	6	0	5	5	2
Mild OSAS	M	6	2	6	3	2
	F	0	1	4	0	1
RERA	M	23	1	17	0	
	F	20	0	9	1	1
Snorer	M	5	0	22	2	4
	F	5	0	10	3	2
	Total	111	29	127	24	

Table 3.
Global assessment.

	N	AI	N	AHI	N	$SpO_2 < 90\%$
Severe OSAS		Mean ± SD				
Preop	20	31.42 ± 16.34	20	57.49 ± 21.85	20	8.01 ± 7.01
Postop	20	16.68 ± 14.17	20	31.89 ± 26.02	20	2.61 ± 23.83
Moderate OSAS						
Preop	10	10.04 ± 4.77	10	3.69 ± 4.13	10	14.92 ± 10.24
Postop	10	20.2 ± 6.08	10	6.73 ± 5.33	10	2.27 ± 2.93
Mild OSAS						
Preop	3	10.1 ± 6.88	3	2.43 ± 3.44	3	8.47 ± 5.83
Postop	3	17.63 ± 5.60	3	2.73 ± 2.27	3	2.67 ± 4.44

Table 4.
Effect of NS on PSG parameters in patients with OSAS.

In the 20 severe OSAS patients the AI, AHI and $SpO_2 < 90\%$ were significantly improved ($p = 0.0002$, $p = 0.0124$, and $p = 0.0015$, respectively). In the 10 moderate OSAS patients, the AI and $SpO_2 < 90\%$ were significantly improved ($p = 0.0051$ and $p = 0.0125$, respectively); however, the AHI was not significantly changed ($p = 0.1394$). In the 3 mild OSAS patients, the AI and $SpO_2 < 90\%$ were significantly improved ($p = 0.0051$ and $p = 0.0125$, respectively); however, the AHI was not significantly changed ($p = 0.1394$).

5. Discussion

A low-invasiveness technique is ideal for surgery. In the present study, the nasal operation showed high efficacy in ameliorating OSAS, hypersomnia, and snoring. A number of patients suffering from hypersomnia and snoring cannot undergo nasal CPAP either for financial reasons or due to the fact that this treatment for CPAP is not covered by the Japanese National Health Insurance System. Our low-invasiveness nasal operation is useful for reducing nocturnal pharyngeal negative pressure, thereby resulting in the amelioration of hypersomnia and/or socially unacceptable snoring.

To our knowledge, this is the first report regarding SDB, including OSAS, in which the nasal resistance was measured in consideration of its pathophysiological importance. Recent studies have found that nasal operations were effective in relieving snoring [6] and ameliorating nasal obstruction, which has consequently increased CPAP tolerance and compliance [7]. The degree of nasal resistance before starting CPAP treatment has a significant effect on the acceptance of CPAP by patients, as a high nasal resistance disturbs CPAP performance [8]. The improvement of the Epworth Sleepiness Scale (ESS) was more significant in the operated group than in the CPAP group [9], although CPAP was observed to ameliorates daytime sleepiness. Robust evidence supports the efficacy of nasal surgery on improving snoring, the subjective sleep quality, daytime sleepiness, sleep-related QOL measures, and other important OSAS outcomes [10]. In patients with chronic rhinosinusitis with polyps, functional endoscopic sinus surgery was shown to significantly ameliorate the sleep pattern and sleep quality [11]. Both the AHI and ESS significantly improved after isolated nasal surgery, but the improvement in the AHI was slightly more significant [12]. Nasal surgery can also effectively improve the subjective symptoms of patients with simple snoring accompanied by nasal blockage as well as those of patients with OSAS [13]. Surgical treatment of nasal obstruction has been shown to improve SDB as well as CPAP. CPAP is considered to be the first line of therapy, but long-term compliance is only about 40%, often because of problems associated with nasal obstruction [14]. Therefore, nasal surgery to reduce nasal resistance during sleep is desirable before starting CPAP. Nasal surgery improved the OSAS severity as measured by PSG, subjective complaints, and three-dimensional reconstructed computed tomography scans [15]. This operation is a cost-effective strategy for improving CPAP compliance in OSAS patients with nasal obstruction [16], although the optimum operative techniques have not been studied. Nasal dilators have shown efficacy in improving nasal breathing but not in improving obstructive sleep apnea outcomes [17], suggesting a need for nasal surgery.

Nasal septum deviation should be investigated in patients with sleep disorders [18]. The most frequent cause of impaired nasal patency was nasal septal deviation, which was found in 82.5% of the patients, including 45% with unilateral impaired patency and 37.5% with bilateral nasal patency [19]. According to our previous study on nasal resistance, even unilateral high resistance affects SDB [4]. Our nasal operation involves septoplasty, submucosal inferior turbinectomy and posterior nasal neurectomy. Measurement of the nasal resistance has proven useful for the treatment of OSAS [20], although the technique used in the cited study was different from that used in ours. Chronic rhinosinusitis (CRS) patients have been shown to have a high prevalence of OSAS, and OSAS symptoms are worse in CRS patients than in others [21].

Nasal surgery alone was partially effective in improving the sleep quality and snoring, but it had no effect on obstructive apnea in patients with OSAS and nasal obstruction [22].

The present study underscored the utility of nasal surgery consisted of septoplasty, submucosal inferior turbinectomy to enlarge the nasal cavity, and nasal parasympathetic nerve resection to achieve a nocturnal low nasal resistance for the amelioration of SDB.

Acknowledgements

We thank T. Yamamoto for his helpful assistance with the statistical analysis.

Conflict of interest

No conflicts of interest and no financial support.

Abbreviation

CPAP	transnasal continuous positive airpressure
SDB	sleep disordered breathing
PSG	polysomnography
ESS	Epworth Sleepiness Scale

Author details

Ken-ichi Hisamatsu[1*], Hiroumi Matsuzaki[2], Itsuhiro Kudou[2] and Kiyoshi Makiyama[2]

1 Tsuchiura Snoring and Sleep-Disordered Breathing Center, Tsuchiura City, Ibaraki Prefecture, Japan

2 Department of Otorhinolaryngology, Head and Neck Surgery, Nihon University Hospital, Chiyoda-ku, Tokyo, Japan

*Address all correspondence to: kenhisam@jcom.home.ne.jp

References

[1] Nilsen AH, Helvik AS, Thorstensen WM, et al. A comparison of symptoms and quality of life before and after nasal septoplasty and radiofrequency therapy of the inferior turbinate. BMC Ear, Nose and Throat Disorders. 2018;**18**:2

[2] Sleep-related breathing disorders in adults: Recommendations for syndrome definition and measurement techniques in clinical research. The Report of an American Academy of Sleep Medicine Task Force. Sleep. 1999;**22**:667-689

[3] Kobayashi T, Hyodo M, Nakamura K, et al. Resection of peripheral branches of the posterior nasal nerve compared to conventional posterior neurectomy in severe allergic rhinitis. Auris Nasus Larynx. 2012;**39**:593-596

[4] Hisamatsu K-i, Kudou I, Takane T, et al. Evaluation of endnasal rhinoplasty for sleep-disordered breathing due to nasal resistance. Practica oto-Rhino-Laryngologica. 2012;**105**:851-857

[5] Johns MW. A new method for measuring daytime sleepiness: The Epworth sleepiness scale. Sleep. 1991;**14**:540-545

[6] Fairbanks DN. Effect of nasal surgery on snoring. Southern Medical Journal. 1985;**78**:268-270

[7] Awad MI, Kacker A. Nasal Obstruction Considerations in Sleep Apnea. Otolaryngologic Clinics of North America. Oct, 2018;**5**(51):1003-1009. DOI: 10.1016/j.otc.2018

[8] Sugiura T, Noda A, Nakata S, et al. Influence of nasal resistance on initial acceptance of continuous positive airway pressure in treatment for obstructive sleep apnea syndrome. Respiration. 2007;**74**:56-60

[9] Tagaya M, Otake H, Suzuki K, et al. The comparison of nasal surgery and CPAP on daytime sleepiness in patients with OSAS. Rhinology. 2017;**55**:269-273

[10] Johnson DM, Soose RJ. Updated nasal surgery for obstructive sleep apnea. Advances in Oto-Rhino-Laryngology. 2017;**80**:66-73

[11] Uz U, Gunhan K, Yilmaz H, et al. The evaluation of pattern and quality of sleep in patients with chronic rhinosinusitis with nasal polyps. Auris Nasus Larynx. 2017;**44**:708-712

[12] Wu J, Zhao G, Li Y, et al. Apnea-hypopnea index decreased significantly after nasal surgery for obstructive sleep apnea: A meta-analysis. Medicine (Baltimore). 2017;**96**:e6008

[13] Wu J, Zang HR, Wang T, et al. Evaluation of the subjective efficacy of nasal surgery. The Journal of Laryngology and Otology. 2017;**131**:37-43

[14] Mickelson SA. Nasal surgery for obstructive sleep apnea syndrome. Otolaryngologic Clinics of North America. 2016;**49**:1373-1381

[15] Cui DM, Han DM, Nicolas B, et al. Three-dimensional evaluation of nasal surgery in patients with obstructive sleep apnea. Chinese Medical Journal. 2016;**129**:651-656

[16] Kempfle JS, BuSaba NY, Dobrowski JM, et al. A cost-effectiveness analysis of nasal surgery to increase continuous positive airway pressure adherence in sleep apnea patients with nasal obstruction. Laryngoscope. 2017;**127**:977-983

[17] Camacho M, Malu OO, Kram YA, et al. Nasal dilators (Breathe Right Strips and NoZovent) for snoring and OSA: A systematic review and meta-analysis. BMC Pulmonary Medicine. 2016;**2016**:4841310

[18] Kara M, Erdogan H, Guclu O, et al. Evaluation of sleep quality in patients with nasal septal deviation via the Pittsburgh Sleep Quality Index. The Journal of Craniofacial Surgery. 2016;**27**:1738-1740

[19] Michalska J, Olszewski J. Polysomnographic evaluation of sleep apnea in patients with unilateral or bilateral impaired nasal patency. Otolaryngologia Polska. 2016;**70**:31-37

[20] Hueto J, Santaolalla F, Sanchez-Del-Rey A, et al. Usefulness of rhinomanometry in the identification and treatment of patients with obstructive sleep apnoea: An algorithm for predicting the relationship between nasal resistance and continuous positive airway pressure. A retrospective study. Clinical Otolaryngology. 2016;**41**:750-757

[21] Jiang RS, Liang KL, Hsin CH, et al. The impact of chronic rhinosinusitis on sleep-disordered breathing. Rhinology. 2016;**54**:75-79

[22] Choi JH, Kim EJ, Kim YS, et al. Effectiveness of nasal surgery alone on sleep quality, architecture, position, and sleep-disordered breathing in obstructive sleep apnea syndrome with nasal obstruction. American Journal of Rhinology & Allergy. 2011;**25**:338-341

Chapter 7

Rhinoplasty in Context of Head and Neck Malignancy

Norhafiza Mat Lazim, Giacomo Spinato and Paolo Boscolo Rizzo

Abstract

Head and neck tumors comprise of multiple epithelial and solid tumors which include nasal cavity and paranasal sinus tumors. Occasionally, the surgical treatment strategy incorporates rhinoplasty procedure in order to achieve better tumor control, preserve function, and attain better cosmetic outcomes. The rhinoplasty is mainly involved with the surgical procedures that intervene with the nasal structure in order to improve the function of the nose along with optimal cosmetic objective acquisition. Multiple surgical procedures and approaches have been introduced in the past decades in refining techniques of rhinoplasty, and it continues to evolve. Most of the times, the procedure is combined with usage of synthetic products, grafts, and biomaterials, in order to ascertain the best outcomes for each of these procedures. In the head and neck oncology arena, rhinoplasty is often performed in combination with other surgical procedures, and it is mainly to improve patient's nasal and sinus functions and cosmesis as well as to enhance quality of life of any given head and neck patients.

Keywords: rhinoplasty, head and neck tumors, surgical oncology, nasal cavity and paranasal sinus tumors

1. Introduction

Head and neck cancer treatment almost always involves some surgical excision of the vital vascularized tissues. In the head and neck region especially, tissue resection will produce significant scarring and esthetic impairment apart from its impact on patient function such as speech, swallowing, breathing, and mastication. In the head and neck surgery, rhinoplasty continues to be among the most popular esthetic surgical treatments at the majority of ear, nose, and throat (ENT) center around the world. This is in fact a reflection of the significance of nose shapes in sociocultural, ethnic, and psychological contexts in the community. In addition and importantly, the nose as a Goldfarb et part of anterior facial skeleton is exposed to multiple insults mainly the trauma, as well as tumors with consequent bony and soft tissue injuries that can have detrimental effects on its sufferers.

Rhinoplasty is a common plastic surgery addressing the anatomical deformity of the nose and aimed at improving nasal function especially the breathing function. It is almost always combined with septoplasty that addresses the nasal septal deviation. There are several indications for septoplasty which include a humpy nose. In order to perform a safe rhinoplasty procedure, a sound knowledge about the nasal anatomy, paranasal sinuses, and its surrounding structures is a must. Treating surgeons and involved team need to be able to know the detail structures of the nasal cavity especially the cartilaginous framework, vascular blood, and neural supply and detail anatomy of facial skeleton as well as the adjacent maxillary and ethmoid sinus structures.

Some of the procedures that were used in esthetic rhinoplasty may also be used in combination with reconstructive nasal surgery in order to achieve free surgical margin or safety margin but, at the same time, to achieve an acceptable esthetic and functional outcome. The goal of any nasal reconstruction surgery is to restore normal nasal shape and function. The essence of nasal reconstruction surgery begins with creating a stable framework. In addition, similar with any other surgical procedures, rhinoplasty carries several significant complications ranging from bleeding, infectious, traumatic, functional, and aesthetic complications (**Figures 1–3**).

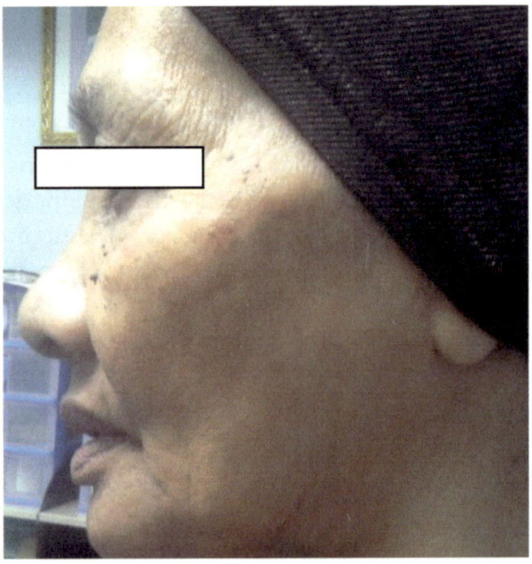

Figure 1.
Lateral projection of the nasal framework.

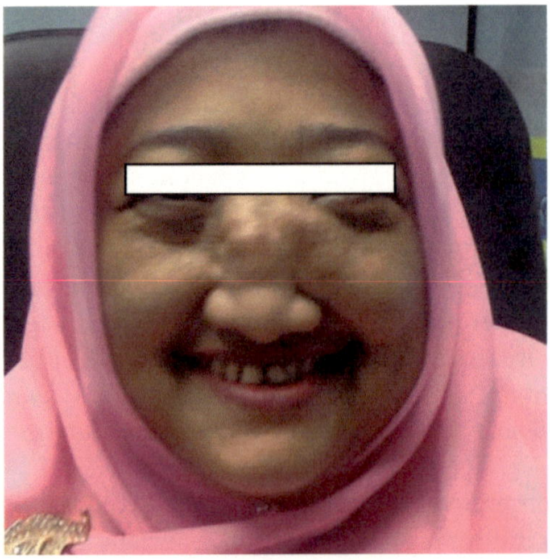

Figure 2.
Anterior profile of the nose with tumor on the nasal bridge.

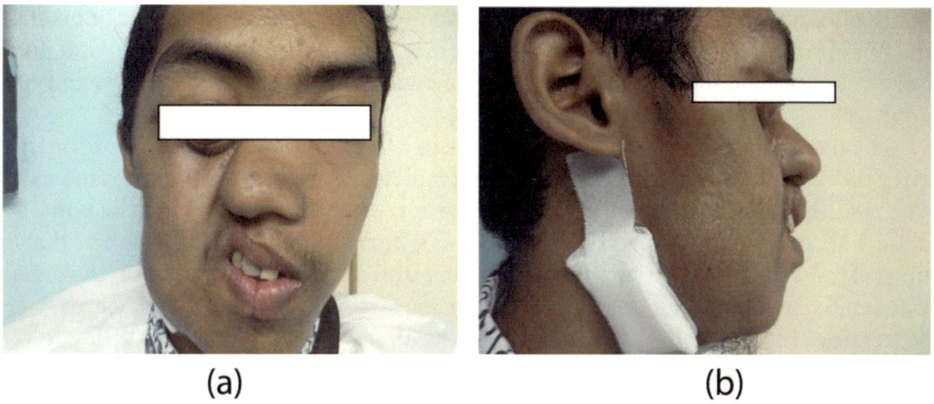

Figure 3.
(a, b): Complications from tumor and its treatment.

2. Anatomical profile of the nose

3. Types of rhinoplasty and its procedure

Over the centuries many anatomists, physiologists, physicists, and surgeons have contributed to the development of rhinoplasty knowledge and techniques. Historically, nasal surgery underwent more development over the years as the nose was frequently the target of mutilation in war conflicts. The first documented case is dated around the year 1000 AD, where *Sushruta*, father of Indian surgery, performed a reconstruction of a mutilated nasal pyramid using pedicle flaps from the cheek and forehead. Several of Indian surgical techniques following the Arab expansion were widespread in the West. They were introduced in Italy first in the mid-1400s and subsequently in the whole Europe [1]. In 1579, Gaspare Tagliacozzi of Bologna described in the *De Curtorum Chirurgia per Insitionem* the reconstruction of the nasal pyramid through the pedicle skin flap of the forearm [2]. In 1881, Karl von Grafe of Berlin coined the term "rhinoplastik" by comparing and describing the various surgical techniques in Europe. It was however because of the development of the front mirror in 1845 and to the introduction of the anterior and posterior rhinoscopy that the physics of air flow was applied to the surgery of the septum. In 1847, P. Heylen first described a septal resection after bilateral dissection of the mucosa, and later Gustav Killian in 1899 modified this technique to prevent the sagging and retraction of the nose [1].

In reconstructive rhinoplasty, it is important to associate the best esthetic result with an efficient airway patency in order to improve quality of life and surgical success. To plan an effective rhinoplasty even under the functional aspect, it is necessary to mention some principles of physiology of the nasal cavity. According to the Bernoulli principle, the inspired air velocity increases in speed in the narrower nasal regions such as the nasal valve or the head of the turbinates, where there is considerable air resistance and where the laminar airflow can increase so as to exceed the number of Reynolds creating vortices [3]. Furthermore, an increase of speed at the level of the constrictions can lead to a decrease in the air pressure to be negative and generate an inspiratory collapse at the level of the lateral nasal wall based on the Venturi effect. These principles of physics, applied to the physiology of nasal breathing, are the basis of functional success in reconstructive rhinoplasty [4]. There is no absolute standard for esthetic proportion of the face. This differs depending on sex, age, body type, and facial characteristics. The female nose is relatively smaller, the dorsum and lobule narrower, than that of the male. In profile, the female dorsum may show a slight concavity, while in the male dorsum, a slight convexity is acceptable. All of these cofactors will influence the final design and approach for the rhinoplasty procedures [5].

The nasolabial angle should be less acute in osteotomy, and formation of the tip after the underlying bony or cartilaginous framework, or both, had been removed. The resulting open-roof deformity had to be corrected by osteotomy of the bony nasal wall and the tip shaped by excision and suturing, including insertion of the tip graft and columellar strut graft. After this, and narrowing of the nose, the defect was smaller and could be closed with local tissue without tension. There were no deformities in the contour, and patency of the airway was maintained. Although the margin of safety was increased, shaping the nasal framework reduced the size of the defect, which allowed tension-free closure with a local flap. The function is guaranteed by trying to recreate the normal anatomy [6, 7]. To obtain a correct morphological and functional rhinoplasty, the procedure may involve different techniques and approaches. The various techniques involve the modification and reconstruction of various nasal subassemblies which are septal, nasal pyramid, nasal vestibule, tip, and turbinate surgery. The sequence of surgical times in reconstructive morpho-functional surgery must bear in mind the pathology and the patient's history and the surgical purposes [8, 9].

Correction of the nasal septum is the basis of functional reconstructive surgery. A septal alteration is the main cause of nasal dysventilation and a cause of deformity of the osteocartilaginous pyramid. The sequence of surgical steps depends primarily whether the endonasal or open surgical approach is used. The endonasal approach involves the mobilization and repositioning of the septum, followed by the correction of the bone pyramid and cartilage with possible osteotomies and additional stabilization surgery of the septum, and finally the modification of the wing of the nose according to the esthetics of the new pyramid. The open approach on the other hand requires the exposure of the wing structures of the nose and the vestibule and of the cartilaginous spine with the mobilization and the repositioning of the septum and the correction of the osteocartilaginous pyramid for the reconstruction of the structure with the modification of the nasal wing [10–12].

The septal reconstructive approach is mostly endonasal. The septum is approached by subperichondrial and subperiosteal dissection, and irreversibly deviating portions are resected. Subsequently, the skin of the osteocartilaginous pyramid is detached by means of a bilateral intercartilaginous incision. Correction of the cartilaginous osteopyramid and possible repositioning depend on the pathology. If appropriate, osteotomies are performed in combination with the monolateral or bilateral wedge resection of the pyramid with its repositioning on the midline. As a last phase of intervention, the nasal wings are harmonized and corrected according to the pathology and the preference of the surgeon. In the external approach, an inverted trans-columellar V incision and a bilateral intracartilaginous incision are performed [13, 14]. The skin is detached from medial crura, dome, and lateral crura. The caudal end of the septum is exposed to the cartilaginous spine. Septal subperichondrial dissection and possible chondrocyte and deviated septal removals are performed. Pyramid plastic and a modification of the nasal valve are similar to endonasal surgery. To correct a deformity of the nasal bone or cartilaginous pyramid, it is possible to perform different procedures such as the repositioning of the anterior septum; the narrowing and push-up of the bone pyramid after osteotomy; the enlargement of the pyramid by inserting a dorsal transplant of septal cartilage, auricular or costal; the increase of the lobular projection; and the narrowing of the lobule itself or the lengthening or lowering of the columella [15–18].

In the case of reconstructions of large defects, it is necessary to use an implant. An ideal transplant must be well-tolerated, without causing any pathologies, not showing any signs of absorption or rejection or altering over time. In literature there are many types of implants and materials utilized over the years. In the nineteenth century, there was an extensive use of gold and silver in the reconstruction of the nose, subsequently using ivory cellulose paraffin and in the 1900s stainless steel. Biological tissues included processed allogeneic or autogenous tissues such as the iliac crest, the tibia, and the auricular costal cartilage. The main disadvantage of biologics is the tendency to reabsorb and deform. The use of non-biological implants instead guarantees the advantages of easy availability; however, if they are not integrated into the nasal tissues, they can lead to possible short- or long-term infections or rejection. Immunological reactions, tissue migration, and carcinogenesis are also described [11, 16, 19–21].

4. Reconstruction technique for rhinoplasty

Proper treatment planning is essential for providing the patient with the best chance of cure and an optimal esthetic outcome. The treatment plan has to be discussed with the patient and immediate relative members in order to ensure their understanding about the whole surgical process and to meet with their expectations. In addition, this is also vital to highlight the expected complications that can arise from the procedures, in order to avoid a cumbersome litigation cases.

The nasal framework is a vital component to be addressed during any rhinoplasty. Regardless of flap used, the supporting structure was the most critical element for the three-dimensional shape of the reconstructed nose. As one of the three elements of nasal reconstruction, frameworks deserve adequate attention during such reconstruction process.

Several approaches have been advocated to decrease postoperative edema and ecchymosis such as performing lateral osteotomies with an angulated saw through an intercartilaginous incision. This technique has been widely described. Other techniques include a modification of Diamond's perforating osteotomy technique, using a 4-mm osteotome, resulting in milder ecchymosis and edema, which was described by Goldfarb et al, as stated in Tahamiler, 2008. Other small techniques but effective are placing drains in the lateral osteotomy incisions allowing blood and serum to escape from the area and reducing the ecchymosis in the periorbital area [22].

Dorsal augmentation is a challenging task for rhinoplasty surgeons in Asia because the required amount of augmentation is frequently substantial. Autologous materials, such as rib cartilages, diced cartilages wrapped in fascia, and dermis or dermofat grafts, are used for dorsal augmentation by many Asian surgeons. Silicone augmentation, however, is still the dominant practice in Asian countries. Alloplastic implants have advantages over autologous materials, such as ease of use, unlimited supply of volume, less invasive nature of the procedure, and incomparably superior esthetic outcomes [23].

There are some technical difficulties and nuances in Asian rhinoplasty; techniques that are highly successful in Caucasian noses are frequently insufficient or unsatisfactory in Asians. Small lower lateral cartilages with short medial crura covered with thick skin make sculpting or suturing tip difficult in Asian population [23].

The use of rib cartilage is related to chest scarring, possible pneumothorax, prolonged operation time, and high emotional or economic burden on the patient. The rigid immobile tip of rib cartilage is often odd and unpleasing. Also, rib cartilage is not immune to complications. Warping and resorption are frequent, and although infection is uncommon, it is possible. Because of its solid nature, it may get fractured with trauma more easily than elastic alloplastic implants. In this regard, rib cartilages are reserved as a last resort rather than as a primary choice for primary esthetic rhinoplasty by many surgeons. The use of rib cartilage in a primary esthetic rhinoplasty should be evaluated carefully on the benefits and costs, patient's comfort level, and possibility of overtreatment [23].

Ideally, the proposed lateral osteotomy pathway should be injected with 1% lidocaine and 1:000,000 epinephrine at least 15 minutes before creating the bony cuts. This will provide a reduction in ecchymosis and bleeding associated with trauma of fracture. Another important consideration is to preserve as much of the periosteum as possible. In the case of lateral osteotomy, this is especially important. Micro-osteotomy using a 2-mm, V-shaped osteotome is recommended because it provides minimal laceration, bleeding, and scarring of the periosteum and subcutaneous tissue. During the course of a lateral osteotomy, the osteotome might accidentally slide sideways, damaging the angular vessels and causing more edema and ecchymosis. The 2-mm, V-shaped osteotome is inserted through the soft tissue to the bone at the piriform aperture. After proceeding cephalically, the osteotome does not slide sideways but glides through the bone where it meets the medial oblique osteotomy [22].

The L-shaped silicone implant has been widely used in Asian countries. One of the major advantages of this silicone implant is a smooth and undisrupted nasal dorsal contour from radix to nasal tip. With the L-shaped silicone implant, augmentation of both the nasal dorsum and the tip is accomplished concurrently without complicated tip procedures. The L-shaped silicone may be an attractive choice for Asian patients because of extreme difficulties of tip plasty in the Asian patient with weak septum, small and weak cartilaginous framework with short medial crura, and thick soft tissue envelope [23].

5. Complications of rhinoplasty

The knowledge of complications in rhinoplasty and nasal reconstruction techniques is fundamental to avoid their formation and also to manage the origin of the complications themselves. Postoperative deformities and breathing dysfunction are the most common complications in rhinoplasty. Tahamiler et al. described additional complications including injury to the lacrimal apparatus resulting in epiphora, the "rocker" phenomenon, the "staircase" phenomenon, hematoma, edema, and ecchymosis secondary to the trauma of osteotomy. Several of these complications were also associated to lateral osteotomies [22].

Many complications could be avoided with a thorough preoperative analysis, in-depth preoperative discussion with the patient, good vasoconstriction, and conservative surgery with possible and careful postoperative monitoring. Some authors recommend not only recording the patient's physical examination and medical history but also discussing the case with the patient himself. This collection will have a fundamental value for any subsequent medical-legal problems [24]. Trying to reconstruct a normal anatomy instead of creating a new anatomy for the patient and to consider a second operation in case of important interventions is crucial in any rhinoplasty case. In general, meticulous attention to detail in the operating room and in the postoperative period is paramount in order to attain success in rhinoplasty. Nevertheless, both complications and suboptimal results do occur even in experienced hands [4, 6].

Among these complications, it is well known that postoperative edema and ecchymosis have been a persistent problem since the advent of rhinoplasty surgery. Periorbital swelling and discoloration are the most distressing to the patients who 24 hours postoperatively may have difficulty with vision because of the edema and is quite self-conscious about esthetic appearance. In a standard rhinoplasty operation, lateral osteotomies are responsible for a significant amount of periorbital swelling and ecchymosis because of the injury of the angular vessels that cross the osteotomy sites and the trauma of infracturing [24]. Complications can be mainly distinguished in cutaneous, infections, intranasal complications, incision complications, hematomas, complications of osteotomies, complications of wing surgery, and complication of transplants. We will venture to examine each of these elements [3, 8, 10, 25].

Skin complications may be linked to cutaneous ischemia due to inadequate skin dissection or due to excessive implant placement or incorrect postoperative bandage. The treatment is to keep a surface as clean and dry as possible in order to prevent infections and possible planning of a revision surgery if the alteration remains conspicuous [20]. Adverse reactions to sutures can cause reactive granulomas and impaired scarring. In case of repeated interventions, telangiectasias can form on the skin of the nasal bridge, and the therapy is cosmetic or in some cases laser. Depending on the type of reconstruction and the choice of the donor flap, skin discoloration may occur. The complications associated with incision design can lead to external scars with serious esthetic consequences, while the internal ones can create important respiratory constructions. The alterations of surgical incisions may depend on the type and number of incisions made, on the inadequate suture of the incisions, on the poor postsurgical control, and on scar infections [16, 26–28].

A very frequent complication after nasal surgery is the nasal and orbital hematomas and ecchymoses. Important in the postsurgery is the evaluation of possible septal hematomas, which, if present, must be drained immediately, and the septal mucosa must be promptly repositioned. To prevent dorsal hematomas, it is important to perform a good, moderately compressive bandage.

Among the infectious complications, there is rhinosinusitis, septal abscess, dorsal abscess, and implant or transplant infection. The abscesses must be promptly drained, while the infection of non-biological implant involves the removal of the same. In case of biological transplant, it is possible to try to conserve it with appropriate intravenous antibiotic therapy [29, 30].

The most common intranasal complications are the synechiae, often asymptomatic. Prevention of synechiae is the placement of a split that prevents contact between the septal mucosa and the side wall. The treatment of the synechiae is the resection of the same after local anesthesia. Septum perforations can cause a variety of complications such as epistaxis crusts, inspiratory whistling, nasal obstruction, and nasal pain. Septal perforations are described with an incidence of between 0.5 and 1% in the hands of skilled surgeons. The most frequent cause of septal perforation is iatrogenic damage, endonasal digital traumatism, bilateral acid burn due to epistaxis, a trauma, cocaine abuse, abscess of the septum, and granulomatous diseases. The anterior and central perforations generally produce more symptoms, while the posterior and basal defects are more elaborate to resolve. The best therapy for septal perforation and prevention ensuring good illumination, a bloodless surgical field, and sufficient surgical exposure is to execute a detachment of the septal mucosa at the subperichondrial level along the correct plane using delicate instruments [31–33].

In the event of a septal laceration, it is important to immediately treat it with stitches if possible.

Therapeutic options for postsurgical septal perforation may be a conservative treatment in the case of an asymptomatic patient, possibly with application of ointments to reduce crusting. Surgical closure of perforation is the best therapeutic option. The success rate of the various techniques can vary depending on the diameter of the perforation. The variables for surgical success are the position and the shape of the perforation, the quality of the Moon margins, and, thus, the presence or absence of cartilage around the defect. In cases of small perforation, a direct closure can be performed by mobilizing and freshening the margins. For wider perforations, rotational flaps or other parts of the septum or nasal floor must be used. Some authors describe the gingival hole flap for large anterior perforations. The septal obturator can be used in case of recurrence of perforation after surgical failure or after extensive demolition in neoplastic patients. Among other complications of septal surgery, there may be sagging of the cartilaginous back which occurs when a high percentage of cartilaginous septum is removed. It can often be associated with retraction of the columella [3, 8, 29].

Among the complications of osteotomies may be an excessive fracture of the sidewall of the bone pyramid which causes esthetic and functional disorders. In order to prevent this complication, an external bandage is important, and the use of glasses in the postoperative period is avoided; in the case of nasal obstruction, the only therapy is surgery. In addition, there may be recurrences of deviations and asymmetries in the event of complete mobilization of the nasal bones or of the septum or in and of the observed detachment of the cutaneous surface or in adequate postoperative protection. In case of resections of osteocartilaginous gibbosities, the open-roof complication can occur [30, 31].

Among the alterations of the nasal wings, there may be the excessive restriction of the lateral crus margin caused by a maneuver to thin the tip or a depressed and flaccid area that can collapse during inspiration with obstruction of the vestibule. With regard to the complications of grafts and implants, these may be mostly occurring late. The most common of the immediate ones are infection, dislocation, and rejection of the graft. To prevent infection, it is important to minimize the risk of ischemia of the skin overlying the transplant and prevent the blood accumulation in the pocket for transplantation with bandages and provide adequate antibiotic coverage. In the event of severe nasal pain and fever, the action patch and any pus secretion from the wound must be removed. The dislocation of the implant can be caused by incorrect positioning or dimensions and insufficient fixation. The use of cartilage as an implant has the highest complication in resorption. In case of infection not treated for a long time, the implant can be extruded. A minimal trauma or infection can be the cause of the expansion of the non-biological implant [33, 34].

6. Application in head and neck malignancy

In head and neck oncology, the free surgical margin is vital in order to prevent any local recurrence and distant metastasis. In the facial region, the bigger the resection, the greater is the defect which consequently causes significant cosmesis embarrassment. Thus, preoperative discussion should be conducted with all team involved in order to come to a consensus for an optimal tumor resection with good margin and thus cause less defect and reconstruction requirement.

An exemplary case includes a 66-year-old lady with history of cystic adenoid mucosal carcinoma of the right nasal septum who had local recurrence staged as T2N0M0 and requires a large nasal excision with amputation of the septum and bony parts of the nose from anterior part to triangular cartilages. In this case the reconstruction was performed in three planes: a musculocutaneous frontal flap for the mucosal plane, a titanium plate for the bone plane, and the nasal skin for the cutaneous plane. Surgical revision with a glabellar flap coverage associated with lipotyping time in unexposed areas improved soft tissue trophicity. Two sessions of complementary lipo-modelings made it possible to obtain a very good and stable coverage. The author concluded that from the oncology point of view, the result is good and no recurrence has been demonstrated with a decline of 10 years and from an esthetic and functional point of view, the results were considered very satisfactory [35].

Skin cancer is an aggressive tumor with high rate of local recurrence. Inadequate treatment will lead to subtotal or total nasal amputation and high morbidity. Basal cell carcinoma (BCC) is the commonest skin type, and the majority is located within the head and neck region where the sun exposure is at the highest. Nearly 90% of cases of BCC is found on the facial region with 30% of cases affecting the nose. Exemplary case is shown in **Figure 4**.

Squamous cell carcinoma on the other hand shows predilection for node metastases. At presentation regional neck nodes are found in 10% of cases. The presence of neck node metastases has major influence on the final outcomes of the diseases. The treatment of this type of tumor involves wide local resection of the tumor in combination with therapeutic neck dissection and/or parotidectomy. **Figure 5** showed a patient with squamous cell carcinoma of the right maxillary sinus with nasal cavity involvement.

The anatomical subsites of the nose that are commonly involved are the ala, nasal tip, lateral nose wall, and nasal dorsum. Primary reconstruction of skin cancer defects is safe in most cases with proper patient selection and reliable histopathological examination techniques. In a large, recurrent, or aggressive skin tumor, the reconstruction should be delayed until more certainty has been obtained than no tumor.

The skin resection defect can be reconstructed and repaired by a variety of techniques which include local skin flaps, septal graft and auricle cartilage, free grafts, and composite graft like skin plus cartilage of conchal. The choice of treatment like in any other type of cancer depends mainly on tumor localization and its extension. For BCC of the nose and nasal cavity, the best treatment option was a radical surgery with safety margin of tumor followed by reconstructive rhinoplasty. Reconstructive rhinoplasty can be done in a staged manner, where a specific procedure is planned at multiple dates, so as to lessen the surgical risk and be able to quantify the desired tissue repair.

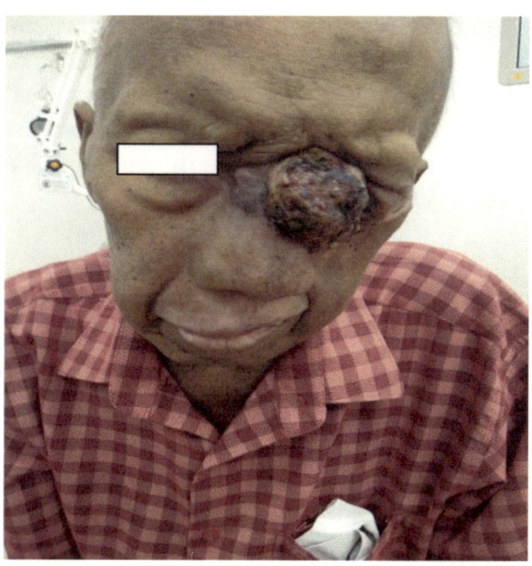

Figure 4.
Basal cell carcinoma of nasal bridge with extension to the medial canthus of left eye.

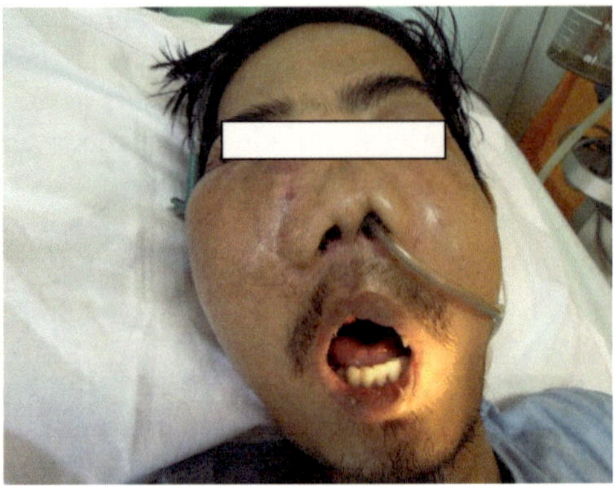

Figure 5.
Squamous cell carcinoma of right maxillary sinus with nasal cavity involvement.

6.1 Revision rhinoplasty

Most of the nasal anatomy alterations found in patient undergoing revision rhinoplasty are challenging to treat, not only from the surgical perspectives but also from psychological point of view. The patients have high expectations and anxieties due to dissatisfaction with previous surgery and difficulty in understanding the limitation of the resurgery cases. In most cases, the need for revision rhinoplasty is the result of a poorly performed prior evaluation, inappropriate patient selection, failure to adequately explain about the limitations related to surgery to the patient, and limitations in performing the surgical maneuvers during the procedure [36].

To optimize patient satisfaction after a revision surgery, the surgeon must be aware of the esthetic and functional complaints reported by the patient, as well as perform a very detailed and objective nasal evaluation, to ensure that no alteration in nasal anatomy goes unnoticed and is amenable to be addressed by surgery. The surgeon must validate the patient's esthetic and functional complaints through a detailed external and internal evaluation of the nose [36].

Complications from revision rhinoplasty is numerous and is based on patient presentation and nasal endoscopy examination; specific complications can be elicited. According to Vian et al., a correlation between subjective obstructive symptoms and the intranasal assessment performed by surgeons was present in 87.5% of cases with one or more nasal obstructive symptoms. Among the patients with respiratory symptoms, the main deformity found was residual septal deviation (56.25%), followed by turbinate hypertrophy and synechiae, both observed in 28.5% of the patients, and the collapse of the internal nasal valve in 19.75% of patients with obstructive nasal complaints [36].

7. Advantages and disadvantages of rhinoplasty and its associated procedures

The advantage of reconstructive technique is to ensure at the oncological radicality good esthetic results with the creation of a new nasal lining, skeletal framework, and skin cover [14, 37]. Ensuring the best esthetic results considers the quality of life of the patients as a whole, initial tumor stage, and functional outcomes [38]. From the literature emerges that surgically reconstructed patients showed a high degree of self-confidence and that prosthetically fitted patients show a high degree of esthetic satisfaction [39]. However, there are no significant differences between patients who received surgical reconstruction and those who received prosthetic rehabilitation after oncological resection.

Although nonsurgical treatment options such as radiotherapy or cryotherapy may be effectively used, surgery is the main treatment option for cancer of the nasal skin. Nasal reconstruction after skin cancer can be very demanding, especially if the patient's expectations are high. Careful assessment of the defect and thorough preoperative planning are as important to the final result as is the technical execution of the procedure [32, 40].

The objective of the reconstruction is not only closing the defect, but closing it appropriately with the optimal flap and in proper with the esthetic subunits. This is the most important point in reconstruction of the nose. During the planning of a nasal reconstruction of adjacent tissue characteristics, the presence of fixed structures and the donor skin area (color, thickness, and laxity) must be assessed. The location and three-dimensional extent of the tumor dictate the choices of repair or reconstruction as well as the timing thereof. Very small lesions can be excised with primary closure or secondary epithelization; other well circumscribed tumors can be excised and the defect closed with an appropriate full-thickness skin grafts and local flaps using one or two stages [33, 37].

Nasal subunits have distinct characteristics; thus, optimal reconstruction should be preferred for each subunit. Nasolabial, cheek, and midline forehead flaps are useful in a variety of instances but usually when less than one-half of the nose has been excised [16]. Advanced nasal skin tumors are not uncommon, and patients who have undergone extended total nasectomies according to many authors are best managed with a prosthesis, as prognosis is often guarded and flap reconstruction may be quite unsatisfactory [41].

For intermediate-sized defects, the choice of reconstruction is usually between skin flap and full-thickness skin graft. For defects on the nose where flap and graft repair may both be technically possible, a flap may be more likely to result in superior cosmetic outcome. Island flap used for ala and back nose reconstruction provides better functional and cosmetic results than the bilobed flap, from both functional and esthetic points of view, but some authors for resurfacing defects following excision of basal cell carcinomas prefer the technique of composite-skin grafting which involves the harvesting of composite-skin graft including the epidermis, dermis, and superficial layers of subcutaneous tissue to obtain the required thickness in the recipient site. The color, texture, and thickness of the composite-skin graft harvested from the preauricular site and the neck compare favorably with the skin of the nose region. Satisfactory results are obtained both clinically and in patient appreciation [15, 33, 42].

Extended resections of nose area require more complex reconstruction methods, including the use of cartilaginous grafts, bony grafts, local flaps, and free flaps [16]. The reconstruction of nasal bone, septum, and esthetically defined units of the nose always represents with certain difficulties. Titanium mesh has been employed as a bone replacement in diverse conditions. As cartilage grafts need a second surgical site, with consequent morbidity, the use of titanium mesh proves useful and safe in the reconstruction of nasal full-thickness defects [19, 37, 43]. In cases of extensive full-thickness resections, free flaps probably represent the most adequate option.

Microsurgical flaps have been proven to be reliable and effective in restoring the missing inner lining elements and adjacent substance losses in total or subtotal nasal reconstruction [16]. Combined with the frontal flap, this esthetic approach allows reconstruction of centrofacial loss of substance layer by layer and facial unit per facial unit. Meticulous attention should be addressed in the artistic rendering of normal nasal dimensions in both size and proportion and form through the use of cartilage grafts and the use of final skin revisions. In addition these techniques help to restore the normal aerial sector [18, 44].

8. Future prospect

Preservation of nasal function and the facial esthetics is a challenging task for every head and neck surgical oncologists as well as plastic reconstructive surgeons around the globe. As many as thousands of head and neck cancer patients, especially the nasal cavity and paranasal sinus cavity tumor, are diagnosed annually, which translates for a need of a better treatment approach and strategy for treating these subsets of head and neck oncology patient in order to maintain the best patients outcomes and improve patient's quality of life. At this juncture, the advancement in the technology and instrumentations has led new discovery and practices that can be implemented at a large scale in fine-tuning the better management protocol for all head and neck oncology patients.

9. Conclusion

Reconstructive nasal surgery must take into consideration multiple factors which include surgeon and patient factors. In order to ensure an excellent quality of life of any treated patient, the surgery and procedure must also re-establish a good nose functionality, reconstructing the normal or near normal breathing, preserving the olfactory perception, and maintaining the ability of heating the breathed-in air. Lesions of the nose are the most challenging for the surgeon, because of the esthetic feature. It mainly aims at achieving good oncological outcomes with good esthetic results. The objective of the reconstruction is not only to fix the defect but to do it appropriately with an optimal flap with crucial consideration of the esthetic subunits. The most important stage of treatment is proper case selection for surgical treatment, selection of optimal reconstruction method that establishes radicalness of resection, and good esthetic and functional results. Many options exist to reconstruct nasal defects that lead to acceptable esthetic results, and at the same time, the surgical reconstruction and prosthetic rehabilitation are available in order to achieve better quality of life.

Author details

Norhafiza Mat Lazim[1*], Giacomo Spinato[2,3] and Paolo Boscolo Rizzo[4]

1 Otorhinolaryngology-Head and Neck Surgery Department, School of Medical Sciences, Universiti Sains Malaysia, Kelantan, Malaysia

2 Department of Neurosciences, Section of Otolaryngology and Regional Centre for Head and Neck Cancer, University of Padova, Treviso, Italy

3 Department of Surgery, Oncology and Gastroenterology, Section of Oncology and Immunology, Universiti of Padova, Padova, Italy

4 Department of Neurosciences, Ear, Nose and Throat, Clinic and Regional Center for Head and Neck Cancer, University of Padua, Treviso Provincial Hospital, Padua, Italy

*Address all correspondence to: norhafiza@usm.my

References

[1] Apostolides PD. Ear Nose and Throat Diseases in Hippocrates. UCL Ear Institute Library historical collection. UCB Pharma; 1997

[2] Spinato G, Boscolo Rizzo P, Tirelli G. History of otorhinolaryngology: From the times of Serenissima till today. In: 11th International SVO Conference on Head & Neck Cancer, Together with Memorial Sloan Kettering Cancer Center (New York) and Mayo Clinic (Scottsdale-Arizona) and GSTTC Gruppo Studi Tumori Testa Collo (Venezia)". Proceedings by Spinato G, Tirelli G, Spinato R. 2014. ISBN: 978-88-85164-39-0

[3] Flanagan P, Eccles R. Spontaneous changes of unilateral nasal airflow in man. A re-examination of the 'nasal cycle'. Acta Oto-Laryngologica. 1997;**117**:590-595

[4] Brunintjes TJD, van Olphen AF, Hillen B. Review of the functional anatomy of the nasal cartilages and muscles. Rhinology. 1996;**34**:66-74

[5] Huzing EH. Incorrect terminology in nasal anatomy and surgery, suggestion for improvement. Rhinology. 2003;**41**:129-133

[6] Stammberger H, Functional Endoscopic Sinus Surgery, the Messerkinger Technique, Mosby Inc; 2000. ISBN 0-941158-969

[7] Rettinger G, O'Connell M. The nasal base in cleft lip rhinoplasty. Facial Pastic Surgery. 2002;**16**:165-178

[8] Daniel RK. Rhinoplasty: An Atlas of Surgical Techniques. New York: Springer; 2002

[9] Cenzi R. Cranio-Maxillo-Facial Rigid Fixation. Clinical Experiences with a New Method. EdiSES srl; 2005. ISBN: 88-7959-183-5

[10] Mang WL. Manual of Aesthetic Surgery. Vol. I. New York-Berlin: Springer; 2002

[11] Papel ID et al. Facial Plastic and Reconstructive Surgery. 2nd ed. Stuttgart-New York: Thieme; 2002

[12] Serra A, Caltabiano R, Spinato G, Gallina S, Caruso S, Rapisarda V, et al. Expression pattern of estroprogestinic receptors in sinonasal inverted papilloma. Oncotarget. 2017;**8**(24):38962-38968. DOI: 10.18632/oncotarget.17161

[13] Meyer R. Secondary Rhinoplasty: Including Reconstruction of the Nose. Springer; 2002

[14] Chiummariello S, Del Torto G, Iera M, Alfano C. The use of local flaps in the one-step nose reconstruction after cancer resection. Annali Italiani di Chirurgia. 2013:84. pii: S2239253X13021233

[15] Monarca C, Rizzo MI, Palmieri A, Fino P, Parisi P, Scuderi N. Island pedicle and bilobed flaps in ala and back nose reconstruction: A prospective comparative analysis. Aesthetic Plastic Surgery. 2012 Oct;**36**(5):1168-1174. DOI: 10.1007/s00266-012-9935-9

[16] Bennett JE, Thurston JB. Cancer of the nose: Ablation and repair. Clinics in Plastic Surgery. 1976;**3**(3):461-469

[17] Huizing EH, de Groot JAM. Functional Reconstructive Nasal Surgery. Verducci Ed. Thieme, second edition. 2006. ISBN 88-7620-736-8

[18] Ayhan M, Gorgu M, Aytug Z, Karantinaci B, Yilmaz E. Comparison of aesthetic outcomes and morbidity of nasal reconstruction with forehead flaps and free flaps. Microsurgery. 2007;**27**(5):411-414

[19] Grajek M, Maciejewski A, Szumniak R, Krakowczyk L. The use of three free flaps in the simultaneous reconstruction of the nose after extensive resection due to malignant cancer. Polski Przeglad Chirurgiczny. 2012;**84**(2):99-101. DOI: 10.2478/v10035-012-0016-1

[20] Tyndorf M, Strzałka A, Kozakiewicz M. Skin cancer of the nose—Methods and results of surgical treatment. Wiadomości Lekarskie. 2016;**69**(2 Pt 2):228-232

[21] Boscolo-Rizzo P, Tirelli G, Mantovani M, Baggio V, Lupato V, Spinato G, et al. Non-endemic locoregionally advanced nasopharyngeal carcinoma: Long-term outcome after induction plus concurrent chemoradiotherapy in everyday clinical practice. European Archives of Oto-Rhino-Laryngology. 2015;**272**(11):3491-3498. DOI: 10.1007/s00405-014-3369-8

[22] Tahamiler R, Erisir F. Lateral osteotomies in rhinoplasty: A safer and less traumatic method. Aesthetic Surgery Journal. 2008;**28**(5):518-520

[23] Kim IS. Augmentation rhinoplasty using silicon implants (review). Facial Plastic Surgery Clinics of North America. 2018;**26**(3):285-293

[24] Spinato G, Cazzato G, Ferlito S, Tirelli G, Boscolo-Rizzo P, Da Mosto MC, et al. Therapeutical innovations and medical responsibility: What's new in otolaryngology. Acta Medica Mediterranea. 2018;**34**:307. DOI: 10.19193/0393-6384_2018_2_49

[25] Tirelli G, Gatto A, Spinato G, Tofanelli M. Surgical treatment of nasal polyposis: A comparison between cutting forceps and microdebrider. American Journal of Rhinology & Allergy. 2013;**27**(6):e202-e206. DOI: 10.2500/ajra.2013.27.3966

[26] Grymer LF. The nasal septum and the development of the midface. Rhinology. 1997;**35**:6-10

[27] Accles R. The nasal cycle in health and disease. Clinical Otolaryngology. 2000;**25**:461-467

[28] Arredondo de Arreola G, Lopez Serna N, Hoyos Parra de R, Salin MA. Morphogenesis of lateral nasal wall from 6 to 36 weeks. Otolaryngology and Head and Neck Surgery. 1996;**114**:54-60

[29] Jayarajan R. A combination flap for nasal defect reconstruction. Annals of Plastic Surgery. 2018;**81**(4):427-432. DOI: 10.1097/SAP.0000000000001483

[30] Salmon PJ, El-Khayat RH. Bridge flap repair for central nasal dorsum defect. The Australasian Journal of Dermatology. 2018;**59**(4):328-329. DOI: 10.1111/ajd.12768. Epub 2018 January 23

[31] Grieco MP, Bertozzi N, Grignaffini E, Raposio E. Nose defects reconstruction with the Zitelli bilobed flap. Giornale Italiano di Dermatologia e Venereologia. 2018;**153**(2):278-282. DOI: 10.23736/S0392-0488.17.05035-0

[32] Zaoui K, Thielen HM, Plath M, Baumann I, Plinkert PK, Federspil PA. Quality of life after nasal cancer resection - surgical versus prosthetic rehabilitation. Rhinology. 2018. DOI: 10.4193/Rhin18.030

[33] Herford AS, Zide MF. Reconstruction of superficial skin cancer defects of the nose. Journal of Oral and Maxillofacial Surgery. 2001;**59**(7):760-767

[34] Carucci JA, Kolenik SA 3rd, Leffell DJ. Human cadaveric allograft for repair of nasal defects after extirpation of basal cell carcinoma by Mohs micrographic surgery. Dermatologic Surgery 2002. 28 (4):340-343.

[35] Aimard R, Lalloue C, Ho Quoc C, Girodet D, Zrounba P, Delay E. Reconstruction of proximal nasal defect after deep carcinological resection, combining titate mesh

with fat grafting. Annales de Chirurgie Plastique et Esthétique. 2017;**62**(2):181-186. DOI: 10.1016/j.anplas.2016.10.002

[36] Vian HNK, Berger CAS, Barra DC, Perin AP. Revision rhinoplasty: Physician-patient aesthetic and functional evaluation. Brazilian Journal of Otorhinolaryngology. 2018;**84**(6):736-743

[37] Broin ES, Naidu ER, Neary P, Edwards G, McHugh M. Reconstruction of major nasal defects. Irish Journal of Medical Science. 1996;**165**(2):125-128

[38] Kline RM. Aesthetic reconstruction of the nose following skin cancer. Clinics in Plastic Surgery. 2004;**31**(1):93-111

[39] Jacobs MA, Christenson LJ, Weaver AL, Appert DL, Phillips PK, Roenigk RK, et al. Clinical outcome of cutaneous flaps versus full-thickness skin grafts after Mohs surgery on the nose. Dermatologic Surgery. 2010;**36**(1):23-30. DOI: 10.1111/j.1524-4725.2009.01360.x

[40] Kaya İ, Uslu M, Apaydın F. Defect reconstruction of the nose after surgery for nonmelanoma skin cancer: Our clinical experience. Turkish Archives of Otorhinolaryngology. 2017;**55**(3):111-118

[41] Gurunluoglu R, Shafighi M, Gardetto A, Piza-Katzer H. Composite skin grafts for basal cell carcinoma defects of the nose. Aesthetic Plastic Surgery. 2003;**27**(4):286-292. Review

[42] Cherubino M, Battaglia P, Turri-Zanoni M, et al. Medial femoral condyle free flap for nasal reconstruction: New technique for full-thickness nasal defects. Plastic and Reconstructive Surgery. Global Open. 2016;**4**(9):e855. DOI: 10.1097/GOX.0000000000000858

[43] Otero-Rivas MM, González-Sixto B, Alonso-Alonso T, Pérez-Bustillo A, Valladares-Narganes LM, Rodríguez-Prieto MÁ. Titanium mesh in reconstructive surgery of the nasal pyramid. Follow-up of our 11 initial cases. International Journal of Dermatology. 2015;**54**(8):961-965. DOI: 10.1111/ijd.12971

[44] Burget GC, Walton RL, B Mole (tranduction francaise). Complete aesthetic reconstruction of nose and adjacent facial units with optimized use of free flaps, cartilaginous grafts and forehead flap combinations. Annales de Chirurgie Plastique et Esthétique. 2009;**54**(6):497-522. DOI: 10.1016/j.anplas.2009.01.036